COURT-ORDERED INSANITY

SOCIAL PROBLEMS AND SOCIAL ISSUES

An Aldine de Gruyter Series of Texts and Monographs

SERIES EDITOR

Joel Best
University of Southern Illinois, Carbondale

Joel Best (*editor*), **Images of Issues: Typifying Contemporary Social Problems**

James A. Holstein, **Court-Ordered Insanity: Interpretive Practice and Involuntary Commitment**

James A. Holstein and Gale Miller (*editors*), **Reconsidering Social Constructionism: Debates in Social Problems Theory**

Gale Miller and James A. Holstein (*editors*), **Constructionist Controversies: Issues in Social Problems Theory**

Philip Jenkins, **Intimate Enemies: Moral Panics in Contemporary Great Britain**

Valerie Jenness, **Making It Work: The Prostitutes' Rights Movement in Perspective**

Stuart A. Kirk and Herb Kutchins, **The Selling of *DSM*: The Rhetoric of Science in Psychiatry**

Bruce Luske, **Mirrors of Madness: Patrolling the Psychic Border**

Dorothy Pawluch, **The New Pediatrics: A Profession in Transition**

William B. Sanders, **Juvenile Gang Violence and Grounded Culture**

Malcolm Spector and John I. Kitsuse, **Constructing Social Problems**

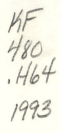

COURT-ORDERED INSANITY

Interpretive Practice and Involuntary Commitment

James A. Holstein

ALDINE DE GRUYTER

New York

About the Author

James A. Holstein is Associate Professor of Sociology, Marquette University. His research brings an ethnomethodologically-informed constructionist perspective to a variety of topics, including mental illness, social problems, family, the life course, and dispute processing.

Dr. Holstein is coeditor of the research annual, *Perspectives on Social Problems*, and coauthor (with J. Gubrium) of *What Is Family?* and *Constructing the Life Course*. In addition, he is coeditor (with Gale Miller) of *Reconsidering Social Constructionism* and *Constructionist Controversies* (both: Aldine de Gruyter, New York).

ALDINE DE GRUYTER
A division of Walter de Gruyter, Inc.
200 Saw Mill River Road
Hawthorne, New York 10532

This publication is printed on acid-free paper ⊗

Library of Congress Cataloging-in-Publication Data

Holstein, James A.
    Court-ordered insanity : interpretive practice and involuntary commitment / James A. Holstein.
        p.   cm. — (Social problems and social issues)
    Includes bibliographical references and index.
    ISBN 0-202-30448-5 (cloth : acid-free paper). — ISBN 0-202-30449-3 (paper : acid-free paper)
    1. Insane—Commitment and detention—United States.   2. Forensic psychiatry—United Sates.   3. Civil procedure—United States.
4. Insanity—Jurisprudence—United States.   5. Deviant behavior—Labeling theory.   I. Title.   II. Series.
KF480.H64   1993
345.73'04—dc20
[347.3054]   92-35481
                                                                        CIP

Manufactured in the United States of America
10 9 8 7 6 5 4 3 2 1

For Suzy

Contents

Acknowledgments

Some close friends and colleagues have suggested that I subtitle this book *They Call Me Bottom Feeder,* not referring to the book's topic, but to the author's intellectual style. Appreciating the constitutive power of categorization, I've resisted, but there is probably a legitimate point to the suggestion. As the proposed title implies, any idea left undeveloped, or any data unanalyzed, in my vicinity is likely to be snatched up, incorporated into my own work. Scavengers have many debts to acknowledge, so this may take longer than an Academy Award acceptance speech.

Jay Gubrium has been a good friend, colleague, and collaborator since I arrived at Marquette University several years ago. I've almost overcome my resentment over his immediate departure for the University of Florida. Working with Jay is a constant effort to keep up, both with the pace of the work and the intellectual development. There is a clear "Gubrian" influence on this project, for which I am deeply grateful.

If Jay pulls me along at at a brisk pace, Gale Miller is always pushing. I'm afraid Gale will never finish all the projects he has lined up for himself, and for us together—despite his religiously followed work schedule that is booked solid for two years past his funeral. Gale is always generous with his time, advice, and assistance, and has contributed much to this project over the years.

I met Bob Emerson and Mel Pollner at precisely the right moment. Having finished graduate school, I wasn't too sure I was interested in doing sociology any more. They kindly and patiently showed me another path, rekindling an interest that was about to expire. While they shouldn't be blamed for what I've done on that path, they are probably responsible for keeping me from wandering aimlessly into another line of work where I might have been able to do some real harm. Mel and Bob have helped and supported this project from the start, and continue to be good friends and major influences.

A number of others have assisted this project in their own ways. Near the beginning, Steve Vandewater patiently explained the importance of looking closely at the organization of ordinary conversation to discover its structuring properties. Beyond that, Steve was always a good colleague, friend, and neighbor. He's the kind of guy who shows up early to help you on moving day, stays to the bitter end, and treats your stuff better than he would his own.

My friend Chris Corey also made his mark on my work. Chris, too, shows up on moving day. He's the kind of guy who, when the manager at the truck rental agency says he just rented out the truck you'd reserved a month ago, grabs the guy by the nose and twists it until the guy discovers that another truck can be ready in just a minute. Over the years, Chris has refused substantive commentary on my work, insisting that it was better because of his neglect. While this probably isn't true, he has contributed in other ways, including taking my wife on her honeymoon, playing center field on my ball team, insisting that I sustain a distinctive "thematic motif" in my writing, and reminding me, both in word and deed, that doing sociology is a lot better than working.

I greatly appreciate the assistance of the following people who have read and commented on various parts of this project: Joel Best, Doni Loseke, Doug Maynard, Joseph Schneider, Carol Warren, and Candace West. Carol's comments over the years have been especially helpful and her review of this manuscript was a great help.

There is a long list of others who have helped and/or encouraged the work that went into this project, some concretely, many of them indirectly: Rick Jones, John Kitsuse, Mike Lynch, Courtney Marlaire, Katie McInnis-Dittrich, Andy Modigliani, Cathy Reszka, Joe Sanders, Manny Schegloff, Norm Sullivan, and Dave Unruh. Of course I must also thank all of the people I studied in the various field sites, especially those I observed in Metropolitan Court.

The project was partially supported by grants from the National Institute of Mental Health (USPHS-MH145830), the National Institute for Handicapped Research (NIHR-G00806802), and the Graduate School at Marquette University.

And now comes the part where I sincerely thank my loving wife for her patience and encouragement. Suzy has more than her share of traditional wifely virtues—sensitivity, compassion, supportiveness, just to name a few. But she has her own interests and agendas, far too many to keep track of mine. To paraphrase an earlier, funnier Woody Allen, it would be a mockery of a travesty of a sham to offer this book as a tribute to marital collaboration. Indeed, Suzy has suggested that I am much too distant, single-minded, and insensitive—I believe she refers to me as a selfish porkface—to do justice to a real marriage. I don't dispute the description, just the degree to which these traits should be seen as faults or virtues. In any case, we often pull in different directions. This book was occasionally one of those pulls. But all in all, it got done, the house is still standing, the family's still together, and we're happy in our own fashion. It might not suit everybody, but I'll take it. The book is for Suzy.

I have discussed some of the materials appearing in this book in other outlets. Related discussions may be found in the following publications: "The Placement of Insanity: Assessments of Grave Disability and Involuntary Commitment Decisions." *Urban Life* (1984) 13:35–62. "Producing Gender Effects on Involuntary Mental Hospitalization." *Social Problems* (1987) 34:141–55. "Mental Illness Assumptions in Civil Commitment Proceedings." *Journal of Contemporary Ethnography* (1987) 16:147–75. "Court Ordered Incompetence: Conversational Organization in Involuntary Commitment Hearings." *Social Problems* (1988) 35:458–73. "Studying 'Family Usage': Family Image and Discourse in Mental Hospitalization Decisions." *Journal of Contemporary Ethnography* (1988) 17:261–84. "Describing Home Care: Discourse and Image in Involuntary Commitment Proceedings." Pp. 209–26 in *The Home Care Experience*, edited by J. Gubrium and A. Sankar. 1990. Newbury Park, CA: Sage. "The Discourse of Age in Involuntary Commitment Proceedings." *Journal of Aging Studies* (1990) 4:111–130. "Producing People: Descriptive Practice in Human Service Work." Pp. 23–39 in *Current Research on Occupations and Professions*, edited by G. Miller. 1992. Greenwich, CT: JAI Press.

Finally, I would like to thank the people at Aldine de Gruyter— especially Richard Koffler, Arlene Perazzini, and Mike Sola—for helping to put this book together.

Introduction

In one of the sites studied for this book, I discovered an eight-page brochure published by the County Community Services Board, titled *Commitment Procedures and Alternatives: Information for Families and Concerned Individuals.* This is its introduction:

> When family or friends are confronted with caring for an individual who has serious mental health problems, many criteria must be considered and decisions made in order to get help for that person. If the person's condition becomes so severe that he or she appears to be dangerous to self or others, or can't take care of basic needs, involuntary commitment may become necessary. If the person is mentally ill . . . and especially if he or she refuses to accept treatment voluntarily, civil commitment may be the most appropriate and even kindest route for loved ones to follow.

The pamphlet offers a sensitive and compassionate synopsis of the purpose of involuntary commitment, a fairly typical view in most communities today. Yet, for all the good intentions supporting the notion of hospitalizing mentally disturbed persons for their own—and the community's—well-being, commitment still represents a massive deprivation of liberty for the committed person. As benevolent as its description might sound, commitment means the loss of many of the everyday rights, opportunities, and responsibilities that most people cherish, yet take for granted. The authority to enforce civil commitment, then, relies on a delicate balance between concern for personal liberty, the state's power to protect individuals who do not seem capable of looking out for themselves, and the state's obligation to ensure the welfare and safety of the community at large.

Public sentiment regarding involuntary commitment seems to vacillate. In the mental health arena, there has been a trend in recent decades toward protecting individual rights—a movement away from a coercive and often inhumane reliance upon enforced hospitalization. Yet, when a person with a history of psychiatric hospitalization makes headlines, say for committing a ghastly crime, cries ring out demanding the community's right to protect itself from the deranged. Support for the use of involuntary hospitalization ebbs and flows, alternating the focus on society or on the individual. Indeed, mental health care generally has undergone "cycles of reform" (Morrissey and Goldman 1984) that have shifted the emphases of treatment and control. In the middle of the twentieth century, for example, publicly supported psychiatric services were provided primarily at state hospitals (Mollica 1983), often against the wishes of those being treated. But the community mental health care movement emerged shortly after World War II, and by the 1970s a sweeping movement to "deinstitutionalize" psychiatric care was under way.

Interest in involuntary commitment has centered on patients' civil rights and the inherent punishment that confinement represents (Hiday 1988). The question has frequently been raised: Is the process fair to those involved? During the 1960s, descriptions of inadequate safeguards for personal liberty and widespread abuses of the legal protections that did exist increasingly undercut the paternalistic stance, stressing the need for due process if persons were to be deprived of their freedom. Studies of commitment proceedings and "lunacy commission hearings" argued that cases were processed too rapidly, there was no real concern for the facts of cases, and legal procedures were all but ignored (Miller and Schwartz 1966; Scheff 1967; Wenger and Fletcher 1969). Some suggested that legal commitment procedures were merely rubber stamps for previously rendered psychiatric recommendations (Miller and Schwartz 1966). Others went farther, claiming that due process was nothing more than an illusion:

> [Commitment] certificates are signed as a matter of course by staff physicians of the Mental Health Clinic after little or no examination. . . . the so-called "examinations" are made on an assembly-line basis, often being completed in two or three minutes, and never taking more than ten minutes. Although psychiatrists agree that it is practically impossible to determine a person's sanity on the basis of such a short and hurried interview, the doctors recommended confinement in 77 percent of the cases. It appears in practice that the alleged-mentally-ill is presumed to be insane and bears the burden of proving his sanity in the few minutes allotted to him. . . . Viewed in this light, the elaborate due process provisions of the Illinois Mental Health Code become a mockery. Nor is this problem native to Illinois alone. (Kutner 1962, p. 86)

Such claims, combined with a growing fiscal conservatism, the development of psychotropic medications that control the symptoms of psychoses, and the general swing toward deinstitutionalization (Benson 1980), have led virtually all U.S. jurisdictions to enact new commitment guidelines and procedures, providing statutory safeguards that limit incursions on individual liberty. With due process rights now protecting persons whose commitment might be sought, today we might ask, Are candidate mental patients still "railroaded" into the psychiatric ward? What are commitment proceedings like under the new circumstances?

Doing the field research for this book, I observed commitment hearings in five different sites across the United States. Most of the hearings were in Metropolitan Court in California, where procedures are fairly typical of what I saw elsewhere. From the inside, Metropolitan Court looks much like any other courtroom. The judge's elevated bench dominates the front of the room, with a witnesses stand to the judge's right and the court clerk's table to his left. Also to the judge's right is a jury box, which was never used for commitment hearings. An attorneys' region occupies the space directly in front of the bench. Lawyers' tables and seats are provided for the representatives of the district attorney's (DA) office, who argue for commitment, and the public defenders (PDs) —or occasional private defense attorneys—who represent those whose commitment is sought. During hearings, the persons being committed sit with their attorneys at the table. These persons have almost always been brought to court from a psychiatric facility, where they have been interviewed, observed, and sometimes treated. Therefore, by the time of most commitment hearings, the person whose commitment is under consideration is already a patient who is technically seeking release.

A low barrier separates the audience area from the participants, and uniformed court bailiffs are always seated near the rail, off to the side. The audience typically includes a variety of observers, mostly witnesses for the hearing in progress, or those awaiting subsequent hearings— usually psychiatrists or other psychiatric personnel—as well as patients awaiting their own hearings. At first glance, one's impression of the court is legal "business as usual," although there is a good deal of traffic in and out of the courtroom, and members of the gallery seem to "speak up" inappropriately more often than typical courtroom decorum permits, addressing the ongoing proceedings, or no one in particular. Overall, the setting seems a little less formal than most courtrooms.

As in other legal venues, the court clerk announces a case, and the principals assemble at the front of the courtroom. The first witness is invariably a psychiatric expert from the facility holding the patient. After some preliminaries, the DA proceeds to the matter at hand, asking the doctor to diagnose the patient's psychiatric condition and offer an opinion about whether commitment is in order. The answers are to the point, professionally framed in psychiatric terminology. And in every commitment case I observed in Metropolitan Court, the doctor said the patient was seriously mentally ill and recommended commitment.

Following direct testimony, the PD cross-examines the witness. There might be a few questions about the doctor's background, or some inquiries about his or her familiarity with the patient. Sometimes the questioning focuses on how well the patient is able to look out for him- or herself—to provide for his or her basic needs. The diagnosis, however, is never directly challenged. The recommendation is another matter, however, as the PD typically probes the bases of the doctor's conclusions, trying to establish that commitment might not be the only resolution to the problem at hand. When the doctor is excused, the DA rests his or her case; the state calls no other witnesses.

The judge now turns to the PD, who almost always calls the patient to testify in his or her own behalf. No controverting psychiatric testimony is offered; no expert or rebuttal witnesses are called. In nearly all cases, the patient is the only one brought to the witness stand to make the case for release. The PD's questions often focus on how the patient feels, how he or she has been doing, or what he or she would do if released. The PD might ask the patient if he or she considers him- or herself mentally ill, and what sort of treatment program he or she would be willing to follow.

Patients' testimony might be best characterized as variable or unpredictable. Much of the time it seems rational, directly responsive to the questions asked. But it often veers to the bizarre, as in a case involving Clarisse Jefferson (CJ):

PD: If you are released, will you take your medication?
CJ: I suppose I will.
PD: Better than you did before?
CJ: I suppose I would. I learned my lesson. I won't let him [referring to her husband] control my mind no more.
PD: Where would you live, Clarisse?
CJ: I'd go back with my husband if I gotta. Live with him and the kids.
PD: Do you think you can manage living with the family?
CJ: Of course. Unless the bastard [the husband] puts the hex on me again.
PD: But you think you could get along all right.
CJ: I suppose I can.
PD: How about living with your mother until things settle down?
CJ: I suppose that would be okay too.
PD: It would mean living apart from your family.
CJ: I could live with it.
[Woman in rear of gallery: You know you could, honey.]
CJ: I know I could. I'll do what it takes. I got enough problems without him cursing me.
PD: Will your mother have a place for you?
CJ: She always does.

When the PD's questions are over, the DA cross-examines the witness. Again, the testimony may combine the routine with the bizarre, but typically all the questions are answered. It is extremely rare for any other witnesses to be called. Occasionally a family member might appear as a witness for the PD, and infrequently social workers or other social service workers might be asked to testify about the circumstances of the patient's life outside the psychiatric facility. After each attorney makes a brief closing argument, the judge considers the possible outcomes, usually remaining on the bench.

Judges freely interject questions into the proceedings at any time, eliciting whatever information might seem necessary. At the close of testimony, the judge might discuss the matters at hand directly with the patient, the testifying psychiatrist, or anyone else whose input might seem relevant. Sometimes the judge questions witnesses who have reoccupied their seats in the audience, or patients who have left the witness stand to sit elsewhere in the courtroom. It is not uncommon for patients to offer their testimony, opinions, or other comments at any time in the proceedings, whether they occupy the witness stand or not.

Finally, the judge renders a decision, either remanding the patient to a psychiatric facility or granting immediate release. The decision is typically explained to the courtroom, and the judge might even offer the patient some "friendly" advice, as he did to Clarisse Jefferson:

> I'm granting the writ [for release], Ms. Jefferson, but I've got to tell you, you stay with your mother and on your medications, or I'll have you right back in the hospital.

Today's commitment hearings are far from the superficial or ritualistic mockeries of justice they were once said to be. Candidates for commitment are represented by counsel and have their cases reviewed by a judge. They can tell their own story and call witnesses to support their claims. The state's claims regarding psychiatric disorder must be based on appropriate diagnostic methods. Proceedings are apparently adversarial, more than perfunctory rubber stamps for psychiatric opinion. But psychiatric judgment remains central to the process. Commitment hearings are not typical legal proceedings either, although the law is always a pressing concern. And, in the cases I observed, there was an approximately equal likelihood that a case would result in commitment or release.

Despite the recent changes—perhaps because of them—the dynamics and outcomes of involuntary commitment hearings are still difficult to fathom. This book tries to understand what goes on in these hearings.

The unique circumstances comprising commitment proceedings raise complex issues relating mental health and illness, law and procedure, and the practical exigencies that arise when persons in the community feel they need to do something about, and for, troubled and troublesome people. In addressing these issues, the book focuses on interpretive practice at the nexus of legal, psychiatric, and practical reasoning. Put most simply, it describes the interactional dynamics through which legally and psychiatrically warranted decisions are publicly argued, negotiated, assembled, and justified.

Within contemporary community mental health care systems, the route to involuntary commitment is often circuitous. The state is now required to seek the least restrictive course of treatment available, making involuntary commitment a generally disapproved alternative, a "last resort" (Warren 1982) for dealing with mental disturbance. With more alternatives available, there is less pressure than in the past to commit mentally ill persons who become problematic. Consequently, to understand who is committed and who is not, or why a particular person ends up in the hospital, requires an analysis that extends beyond commitment proceedings to the interorganizational network that processes psychiatric cases (Warren 1982). Commitment hearings are merely one aspect of the process—albeit one that is extremely consequential for persons whose cases proceed to that point in the process. While the book is mainly about commitment hearings themselves, it takes the wider context into account as it analyzes the interpretive practices through which decisions are produced.

But the book is not simply a description of how facts are presented and laws applied in court. Rather, it analyzes how hearing participants construct and organize arguments that are legally, psychiatrically, and practically accountable. Mental illness is always important to these arguments, but, as I will argue, it is not the deciding criterion in commitment decisions. Rather, commonsense reasoning about everyday competence and the challenges posed by mental illness produces an orientation to the practical side of how candidates for commitment manage their lives. Consequently, commitment proceedings are not mere "lunacy hearings," where sanity is the central issue. Rather, they embody a more holistic orientation to how troubled lives might best be understood and managed, viewing psychiatry, the community, and the law as resources for care and control.

The practical orientation of commitment hearings focuses participants' attention on the relative appropriateness of hospitalization versus noninstitutional accommodations for the person whose commitment is sought. The book argues that commitment decisions orient to the "tenability" of situations that patients pose as alternatives to hospitalization.

The argument throughout is that the features of persons and circumstances that are considered as part of tenability arguments and assessments are interpretively accomplished, constituted in the conversational exchanges that comprise commitment hearings.

Because interactional practice and interpretive context are intertwined in the commitment process, it is difficult to highlight one without implying that the other is of lesser importance. Foregrounding practice necessarily relegates context to the background, and vice versa. In order to stress the importance of each, the book moves back and forth between practice and context, alternately emphasizing each and underscoring their inextricable relation.

Chapter 1 presents the book's theoretical grounding, conceptualizing involuntary commitment proceedings in terms of interpretive practice. Alternative perspectives on mental illness are introduced, and the controversy pitting the psychiatric and labeling models is briefly discussed. As an alternative to these more conventional approaches, the book offers a "constitutive" perspective on mental illness, suggesting how the approach can be used to understand the commitment process.

Chapter 2 briefly reviews the history of confinement of the "mad" or "insane" in America, then brings the discussion up to date by outlining contemporary involuntary commitment laws. It then describes the book's methodological approach.

Chapter 3 takes up the organizational context of commitment proceedings, highlighting background assumptions and orientations that form an interpretive context for decision-making. It outlines the prevailing assumption that all persons whose commitment is being considered are mentally ill, and adumbrates some of the implications of the assumption. It also considers the organizational orientations, interests, and priorities that condition the commitment process.

The interactional organization of commitment proceedings is detailed in Chapter 4. A prototypical "hearing sequence" is described, the interactional framework for articulating the crucial issues of the commitment process. The sequence provides ways for commitment participants to display their orientation to locally relevant legal and psychiatric concerns, as well as to the need to help and control psychiatrically troubled persons.

One of the central issues to be decided in commitment hearings is whether released patients can manage their lives outside the hospital. While all candidates for commitment who advance to the point of commitment hearings are assumed to be mentally ill, their interactional incompetence is not taken for granted. Chapter 5 shows how documents of competence and incompetence are interactionally produced during commitment hearings.

If all persons whose commitment is sought are considered mentally ill, what discriminates between cases? Chapter 6 argues that participants in commitment hearings exhibit an orientation to the tenability of patients' community living circumstances as the basis for their arguments. Tenability is analyzed as a descriptive accomplishment, fashioned by matching patients' needs with the community living accommodations available to them.

While persons are not committed on the basis of mental illness alone, psychiatric condition is still significant to the commitment process. Chapter 7 examines the use of the mental illness assumption as an interpretive framework for assessing commitment-relevant claims, descriptions, and arguments.

Chapter 8 argues that interpretive practice reflects its social and cultural circumstances. It describes the ways that social and organizational location shape commitment arguments, contending that culturally normal forms are used as interpretive resources for describing and evaluating patients and their proposed living circumstances.

The concluding chapter summarizes the book's major themes and examines the implications of understanding commitment decisions in terms of culturally grounded interpretive practice. First, it considers the custodial implications of seeking tenable community accommodations for persons believed to be mentally ill. Then it discusses the accountability structures to which commitment arguments orient. The chapter closes by arguing that commitment proceedings serve to "rationalize" the community's compassion for the mentally ill, while simultaneously "domesticating" its interest in controlling those considered psychiatrically deranged.

While the book is specifically about involuntary commitment proceedings, it is also concerned with aspects of interpretive practice that transcend the settings studied. To that end, it highlights general features of the social processes through which the factual character of objects and experience is established. The analysis emphasizes the situated, interactional production of ordinary features of everyday life—things like deviance and normalcy, competence and incompetence, age and gender, home and family.

Chapter 1

Interpretive Practice and Involuntary Commitment

> We have yet to write the history of that other form of madness, by which men, in an act of sovereign reason, confine their neighbors. . . . To explore it we must renounce the convenience of terminal truths, and never let ourselves be guided by what we may know of madness. None of the concepts of psychopathology, even and especially in the implicit process of retrospections, can play an organizing role. What is constitutive is the action that divides madness, and not the science elaborated once this division is made and calm restored.
>
> —Michel Foucault, *Madness and Civilization*

In his iconoclastic treatise on the relation between *Madness and Civilization*, Michel Foucault (1965) fashioned a radical "archaeology" of the public distinction between "madness" and "reason." Conceding neither objectivity nor immutability to madness, Foucault traced the emergence of cultural categories through the classical age that came to separate reason from nonreason. Madness, he argued, was not the invariant figure known today as mental illness, something misunderstood and poorly recognized in other times. Rather, madness's shifting identity was variously constituted through distinctive frameworks of perception; its recognizable forms were not discoveries of previously obscured truths, but instead represent the development or convergence of alternative socially, culturally, and historically situated discourses. Treating madness not as reality, but as judgment, Foucault described how ascription became "fact"—indeed, the medical, psychological fact of "mental illness" that provides the basis and motivation for modern psychiatry, and in turn reifies the "objective" psychiatric truth of madness.

For Foucault, madness is not an object of knowledge; it is an historically variable way of knowing. His interest lies in how the *concept* of madness was variously constituted in different sociohistorical eras. *Madness and Civilization* is something of a "counter-history" (Cousins and

1

Hussain 1984) to modern chronicles of mental illness and psychiatry, versions sanctioned by the medical model of insanity. In it, Foucault elaborates the varying interpretive conditions that underpin the "action that divides madness" from what it might otherwise be called. His work elucidates the emergence and transformation of the category that some community members have used to sequester others in order to control, reform, discipline, or—today—therapeutically treat them.

Dividing actions are figural for Foucault. *Madness and Civilization* tells us how we came to our modern categorization of madness—mental illness—and how assignment to that category has become the basis for humanitarian internment and therapy, first in asylums, now in psychiatric wards. It specifies a history of a category that is used to differentiate individuals and justify reactions. But the dividing action—the segregation and treatment of "madness"—also involves everyday applications of categories and labels, *mental illness* currently being the most prominent.

This book is about interpretive practice—the procedures through which people represent, organize, and understand reality. It emphasizes the social processes that attach meaning to experience. It treats the interpretive practices implicated in involuntary commitment proceedings as forms of "action that divide," actions that provide the basis for segregation, confinement, and care. In contrast to Foucault's historical interest, the book is concerned with the practical use of *mental illness* and related classifications, focusing on the ways people employ labels, categories, and ascriptions to designate others for special treatment. The analysis does not rely upon Foucault as an historical authority as much as it appreciates his conceptual and methodological approach.

Imprecise estimates suggest that there are between 100,000 and 150,000 persons in the United States receiving inpatient psychiatric treatment against their will (Smith and Meyer 1987). While there is a long history of confining the "insane," reformed mental health legislation currently mandates that involuntary commitment for psychiatric treatment must be both medically and legally warranted, providing procedural safeguards against illegal or unreasonable detention. This book describes the dynamics of commitment proceedings, analyzing the everyday interactional practices that produce legal decisions to hospitalize and treat persons who resist such confinement. It is centrally concerned with how hearing participants interpretively construct and manage legally and psychiatrically accountable findings.

Interpretive practice specifies social problems and their victims; it distinguishes deviance from normalcy. This book is about how persons ascribe and deploy "madness" and its modern-day variants in legally circumscribed ways to "confine their neighbors." It is about the practical reasoning, cultural categories, and interactional comparisons—involving reference to "normal" forms as well as accounts of mental derangement—that are used to accomplish involuntary commitment decisions. And it is about the social, institutional, and legal contingencies that condition and influence those decisions. Its aim is to describe the socially organized dividing practices that separate the involuntarily committed from the rest of us.

Perspectives on Mental Illness

Mental illness provides a rationale for depriving persons of their freedom in order to promote their well-being. While vernacular and technical uses of the term frequently diverge, both psychiatric and common-sense definitions appear in civil commitment statutes and procedures. Definitional matters are central to remedial intervention and hospitalization. *Madness* and terms like it have been applied to diverse behaviors across different historical eras, but, as Foucault (1965) argues, mental illness has not been a singular phenomenon that was simply (mis)understood under a variety of psychiatrically naive guises or labels. Rather, distinctive phenomena—such as madness, possession, insanity, and mental illness—have been constituted by the alternative discourses through which they have been identified and characterized.

Nonetheless, a durable psychiatric model of mental disorder has emerged since the nineteenth century, casting a variety of "abnormal" or culturally "deviant" behaviors, perceptions, and affects as symptoms of a disease that manifests properties similar to those of other physical illnesses. Mental illness has thus become a general designation for a variety of disorders or pathologies of the mind that plague those afflicted. The *Diagnostic and Statistical Manual of Mental Disorders III-R* (1987) of the American Psychiatric Association provides a mechanism for classifying and differentiating disorders for the purpose of identification and treatment, exemplifying the contemporary psychiatric or medical perspective.

Considerable sociological analysis has incorporated versions of the psychiatric model to studies of the etiology, identification, and treatment of mental disorders (see, for example, Hollingshead and Redlich 1958, Kessler and Cleary 1980, Mechanic 1980). The sociological aspect of such work derives from considerations of the social distribution of what is considered to be an objective and observable phenomenon. Since the 1960s, however, an "antipsychiatric" model of mental disorder has also developed, often arguing with sociological overtones that mental illness is not an illness at all. Bateson, Jackson, Haley, and Weakland (1956), for example, suggest that schizophrenia is analyzable as attempts to deal with difficult, "double-binding" communication patterns, while Laing (1967) similarly contends that the "disease" is a form of dissociation from intolerable social circumstances. Adopting an even more sociological position, Szasz (1961) argues that mental illness is a "myth"—an inappropriate metaphor for understanding persons who have difficulty dealing with "problems in living." Mental disorder, he suggests, should be viewed within the framework of a "game-playing model of human behavior," treating mental symptoms as role-playing adaptations to problematic social circumstances.

In his attempt to link "labeling theory" to the study of mental disorder, Scheff (1966) has offered perhaps the most elaborate, explicitly sociological claim for a theory of mental illness. Becker's classic statement of the labeling perspective on deviance, of course, claims that

> deviance is not a quality of the act the person commits, but rather a consequence of the application by others of rules and sanctions to an "offender." The deviant is one to whom that label has been successfully applied; deviant behavior is behavior that people so label. (Becker 1963, p. 9)

Adapting this argument to mental illness, Scheff suggests that the sort of rule breaking or norm violation that invites the label *mental illness* generally involves expectations so fundamental and taken for granted that they are assumed to be standards of natural, decent, understandable behavior. He calls these violations "residual rule breaking." Noting that residual rule breaking is extremely widespread, Scheff asserts that most persons displaying such "symptoms" are never categorized and treated as mentally ill. Consequently, his theory focuses on the social and contingent reasons that some residual rule breakers and not others are designated for the label and role of *mentally ill.*

Academic and professional controversy persists regarding the relative viability and value of the competing perspectives. The psychiatric model is more attentive to etiology, while sociological approaches are more concerned with societal reaction to and control of mental illness. The psychiatric model provides a framework for understanding and treating persons who appear to be severely troubled, while the labeling approach cautions us about the cost of creating and applying deviance categories in order to effect controls or cures—even seemingly benign medical ones. The debate has been acrimonious at times, but it appears to have subsided as the radical antipsychiatry movement's popularity waned in the absence of a viable treatment alternative, while research compatible with the medical model flourished.

This book is not interested in arbitrating the old dispute. Instead, it takes an alternative approach to definitional matters. Its topic is interpretive practice in commitment proceedings, so it is mainly concerned with how persons involved in the proceedings understand, define, interpret, and use the concept of mental illness or psychiatric disorder—along with myriad other interpretive resources—to fashion legal decisions. Accordingly, the *process* of invoking and applying definitions, categories, and practical interpretive procedures is the focus of analysis. The book describes what participants in commitment proceedings say and do about mental illness and involuntary confinement and treatment, what they talk about in the process of their decision-making, and how they use categories—like family, gender, and psychiatric disorders, to name a few—to accomplish their decisions.

The book's approach to mental illness is to treat it as a practical ascription, a category or label that persons in everyday circumstances use to describe behavior, characteristics, or conditions. Rather than assigning a transcendent meaning to the term, the focus is on indigenous usage. The perspective thus conceives mental illness (or, for that matter, any other social phenomenon) in terms of the processes through which it is realized and interpreted—that is, constituted. While conventional labeling theorists ostensibly embrace the proposal that deviant behavior is behavior that people so label, their analyses fail to maintain a radical commitment to construing deviance (or mental illness, or any other characteristic) in terms of those processes through which labels are attached. The constitutive alternative suggests that meaning is not inherent in any particular object, person, or event, but instead is attached through language and interaction. The analytic project from this standpoint is to discern and describe the processes and practices through which persons articulate and assign meanings to make sense of everyday activities, providing their actions with a sense of being orderly and accountable. Following this argument, the book is about interpretive practices—ways of doing things through interaction and discourse—that make up, and make sensible, involuntary commitment proceedings.

Reality as an Interactional Accomplishment

The constitutive approach to mental illness is underpinned by the notion that the "objective reality of social facts" is a socially organized, interactional accomplishment (Garfinkel 1967). Taking the "facts" of social life to be socially constructed, however, runs counter to the way we generally understand the world we inhabit. When we think of the life world (Schutz 1970), we think of a reality that is objective—something "out there," existing apart from the acts of observation, perception and description through which we know it. The meaning of actions and objects seems to be intrinsic to those acts and objects, something self-evident, something everyone knows, or could possibly know. Social interaction in this world seems to be a matter of reacting and responding to reality's inherent meanings—transporting, conveying, and manipulating those meanings. Language is typically considered in terms of its representative function. Words, we believe, merely convey meanings that emanate from the things and acts that the words reference, correspond to, or stand for. According to this conception, interaction helps us navigate reality, while the essential task of language is simple description—telling about reality.

An alternative approach, informed by ethnomethodological (Garfinkel 1967; Heritage 1984; Pollner 1987), social constructionist (Berger and Luckmann 1966), and symbolic interactionist (Blumer 1969) traditions, conceives of everyday realities as interactively constructed and sustained. Challenging reality's objective, "out there" status, the approach suggests that persons' depictions of, and dealings with, their social worlds create or constitute those social worlds as meaningful phenomena. From this perspective, interaction, in general, and, more specifically, talk and language use are not mere ways of conveying meaning. Rather, they are ways of *doing things with words* to produce meaningful realities and formulate the life world. In a sense, the orderly and recognizable features of social circumstances are "talked into being" (Heritage 1984, p. 290) as descriptive practice organizes, manages, and transforms reality.

Descriptions—as when we describe someone as mentally ill, or incompetent, for example—are not disembodied commentaries on ostensibly real states of affairs. Rather, they are constructive *actions*—applications of labels and assignments of meaning—that are consequential within specific situational and interactional contexts. Description is practical, purposeful activity; descriptions are *reality projects.* Viewing reality as a social construction shifts our analytic interest from the objective features of the world per se, to what Pollner calls "worlding" activities—the interpretive work whereby that world and its attendant concerns are assembled and sustained.

Schutz (1964) has stressed that the social world is interpreted in terms of commonsense categories and constructs. These constructs are the resources with which persons interpret their situations of action, grasp the intentions and motivations of others, achieve intersubjective understandings and coordinated actions, and more generally manage the life world. Both natural and social objects are interpretively constituted and continuously updated through interpretive frameworks derived from a socially supplied stock of knowledge at hand. This stock of knowledge—

held in the form of typified constructs and categories—serves as a pragmatic resource for organizing understandings of and actions in the life world. Understanding involuntary commitment proceedings thus requires a focus on participants use of commonsense knowledge and practical reasoning.

Analyzing commonsense knowledge and practical reasoning requires that we "bracket" (Schutz 1962) the social world and our everyday assumptions about its facticity. That is, rather than assume that particular objects or social forms exist, we must suspend belief in their objectivity. Instead we assume that persons interpretively create, assemble, produce, and reproduce the things to which they orient. Our analytic attention can then be focused on the practices, methods, and procedures through which persons produce the sense of social order that sustains their belief in an orderly, objective world. At the same time, we avoid comparisons between commonsense practices and idealized standards that might lead us to point out errors in indigenous, everyday interpretations. By refusing an omniscient position, we resist the temptation to invidiously compare persons' everyday activities to abstract standards, treating those activities instead as artful, reality-producing practices.

This stance amounts to a sort of analytic indifference toward the phenomena being studied (Garfinkel and Sacks 1970). This does not mean we lose interest in the phenomena, or disregard them because they are insubstantial or subjective. To the contrary, it means that we adopt a perspective outside and apart from the objects of our inquiry, allowing us to dispassionately examine the practical activities that constitute those objects, making as few presuppositions as possible. Analytic indifference allows us to discern and describe how everyday actors produce and manage the myriad features of their social lives and worlds without judging their actions against some transcendent standard of what the life world is "really" like.

The Labeling Controversy

A constitutive perspective offers a new outlook on involuntary commitment proceedings. This is not to suggest, however, that conventional analyses have been uninteresting. Indeed, studies of commitment procedures have been at the heart of the most controversial, if not the most important, debate in contemporary psychiatric sociology. During the 1960s and 1970s, labeling theory (Becker 1963) ascended to such stature that some called it the dominant sociological perspective on deviance (Gibbs and Erikson 1975; Gove 1982; Sagarin and Montanino 1976). A set of critiques congenial to the labeling perspective—including work by

Goffman (1961, 1969), Laing and Esterson (1964), Szasz (1961), Rosenhan (1973), and especially Scheff (1966)—challenged the prevailing psychiatric understandings of mental disorder with such vigor that a full-fledged dispute captivated the field for nearly two decades. Galvanized by the clash of perspectives, sociologists argued the relative merits of the psychiatric and societal reaction approaches with uncommon passion.

Thomas Scheff and Walter Gove dominated the controversy. Their exchanges evolved into a large-scale debate that raged across the pages of major sociological publications for well over a decade [see Horwitz (1979) and Gove (1980, 1982)]. At its height, Gove and Scheff commanded center stage in the *American Sociological Review* (Gove 1970, 1975, 1976; Scheff 1974, 1975, 1976) in what was arguably the most rancorous public professional squabble of its time. Unfortunately, the dispute generated more heat than light as arguments and rebuttals mounted. Wearied by the lack of resolution or conceptual progress, Horwitz eventually mocked the exchange as

> [Gove's] rebuttal of Scheff's original position . . . , replies to this rebuttal . . . , rebuttals of these replies . . . , replies to the rebuttals of the replies to the rebuttal . . . , and rebuttals of these as well. (1979, p. 296)

And of course there were numerous commentaries on the resolution, or futility, of the debate (Akers 1972; Horwitz 1979; Imershein and Simons 1976; Krohn and Akers 1977).

The centerpiece of the controversy was Scheff's book, *Being Mentally Ill* (1966). As the most detailed and explicit formulation of the labeling perspective, Scheff's "sociological" or "societal reaction" theory of mental illness provided the springboard for Gove's assault on the perspective. To summarize briefly, Scheff argued that "we can categorize most psychiatric symptoms as instances of residual rule-breaking" (1966, p. 33). The culture of a group, he noted, provides a vocabulary of terms for categorizing norm violations like crime, for example. The terms are derived from the types of rules that have been broken and from the type of behavior involved in the norm violation (1966, p. 34). But there are times when no categories seem to fit, instances that represent a "residue of the most diverse kinds of violations for which the culture provides no explicit label" (1966, p. 34)—residual rule-breaking. It is these types of violations that are typically attributed to mental illness. According to Scheff, residual rule-breaking is widespread and frequent; virtually everyone at some time behaves in a fashion that corresponds with the cultural typification of mental illness. The causes of residual deviance are extremely diverse, he argues, and often benign, so that they should not be taken to indicate personal pathology or disorder. Consequently, we should not become preoccupied with finding their causes. Rather, we need to focus on societal reactions to acts of residual deviance to understand how mental illness emerges.

Social reaction, Scheff argued, is the most important factor in stabilizing mental illness (1966, p. 54). To this, Gove replied that one's psychiatric condition and behavior were more important in determining the likelihood of being identified and treated as mentally ill than were nonpsychiatric factors. Scheff's response, of course, was that social contingencies, not psychiatric factors, were the major determinants of whether persons were identified as mentally ill.

Involuntary commitment became central to the debate in part because it provided an opportunity to examine procedures whereby mental illness was determined and reactions to it were formally specified. By casting involuntary hospitalization as a dependent variable, researchers could test hypotheses concerning the relative influence of psychiatric and societal reaction variables on commitment decisions. Scheff, for instance, suggested that psychiatric professionals' predispositions to find pathology and prescribe treatment affected commitment decisions, independent of candidate patients' psychiatric condition. Once a person comes to the psychiatric community's attention on the grounds that he or she is mentally disturbed, he argued, the person will almost certainly be labeled, treated, and hospitalized. This is so because psychiatric personnel are more sensitive to signs of mental illness than the general public and see a wider array of persons as disturbed and in need of care. Guided by a medical ideology, they feel that it is safer to treat someone who may not be mentally ill than it is to fail to treat someone who is.

In a study of judicial hearings to determine if persons should be involuntarily hospitalized, Scheff (1964) found the proceedings to be brief (the mean time for hearings was 1.6 minutes), perfunctory, and insensitive to candidate patients' rights, findings echoed in Miller and Schwartz's (1966) study of commitment proceedings. He also found that psychiatrists conducting psychiatric examinations as part of commitment procedures appeared to presume illness to the extent that they were able to "establish illness even in patients whose appearance and responses were not obviously disordered" (Scheff 1966, p. 139). Scheff thus concluded that the evidence upon which examiners based their decisions seemed arbitrary and the commitment process, in general, seemed predisposed to hospitalize any candidate patient once proceedings had begun.

Proponents of the labeling position also contended that social characteristics and contingencies influenced decisions to commit; in some cases they argued that such factors were more important than psychiatric condition itself. Haney and Michielutte (1968), for example, found that a candidate patient's age, the rate of available psychiatric beds, the

type of person initiating commitment proceedings (family member versus agent of the community), and the composition of the psychiatric
examination committee (psychiatrists versus nonpsychiatrists) affected
commitment decisions. Similarly Haney, Miller, and Michielutte (1969)
found that social characteristics of petitioners for commitment (age, marital status, and occupation) relative to those of candidate patients influenced hearing outcomes. Scheff (1975) argued that a candidate patient's
social class or socioeconomic status influences commitment decision.
Finally, Wenger and Fletcher (1969) found that the presence of a lawyer
to represent the candidate patient was significantly associated with the
likelihood of decisions not to commit, while Wilde (1968) noted that
commitment decisions were associated with characteristics of responses
of others like diligence of the petitioner and identity of decision-makers.

Gove's response to the labeling arguments was unequivocal: "The
available evidence . . . indicates that the societal reaction formulation of
how a person becomes mentally ill is substantially incorrect" (1980b, p.
85). In a series of scathing, if not devastating critiques, he took issue
with the methodological adequacy, as well as the interpretation of, the
empirical results of the studies Scheff and others cited in support of the
labeling position (Gove 1970, 1980b). On the issue of involuntary mental
hospitalization, Gove was adamant that

> a substantial majority of the persons who are hospitalized have a serious
> psychiatric disturbance quite apart from any secondary deviance that
> might be associated with the mentally ill role. Furthermore, persons in the
> community do not view someone as mentally ill if he appears to act in a
> bizarre fashion. On the contrary, they persist in denying mental illness
> until the situation becomes intolerable. Even after prospective patients
> come into contact with public officials, a substantial screening occurs,
> presumably sorting out persons who are being railroaded or who are less
> disturbed. . . . Perhaps the most telling evidence is that, to the extent to
> which individual social attributes do seem to have an effect on the hospi-
> talization process, their effect is in the opposite direction from that posited
> by the labelling perspective—that is, controlling for level of disorder, it is
> the individuals with the most resources who are most likely to enter the
> role of mentally ill. (1980b, p. 85)

The aspect of the Scheff-Gove debate concerned with involuntary
commitment seemed to boil down to a dispute over the relative importance of psychiatric versus nonpsychiatric factors in predicting involuntary commitment. And the issue was allowed to carry at least part of the
burden of deciding the larger contest over the predominance of the
labeling or psychiatric models. Most participants and observers appeared to understand the controversy as a clash between conflicting
visions of mental illness. Scheff (1975, p. 253) for example, suggested

that "the central issue . . . is the relative importance of social system, as against, individual contingencies in labeling," while Gove (1980a, p. 14) countered that "the issue should be the importance of the labeling explanation relative to other explanations . . . which explanation is most powerful, i.e., which accounts for the most variance." In a peculiar fashion, however, the conceptual grounds for the dispute were articulated (or, perhaps more accurately, were vaguely implied) in such a way as to actually blur the distinction between the competing perspectives. And, even more remarkably, almost no one seemed to notice.

Recall that the foundation of Scheff's labeling approach was Becker's (1963, p. 9) radical axiom that "deviance is not a quality of the act the person commits, but rather a consequence of the application by others of rules and sanctions to an 'offender'" (quoted by Scheff 1966, p. 32). Scheff (1966, p. 32) explicitly embraced this position, stating that "the concept of deviance to be used here will follow Becker's usage." Quoting Becker at length, he concluded with Becker's maxim that "the deviant is one to whom the label has successfully been applied; deviant behavior is behavior that people so label" (Scheff 1966, p. 32 citing Becker 1963, p. 9). As Pollner (1974, 1978) has suggested, a "strong" reading of this statement holds deviance to be nothing other than the processes and practices through which persons "orient to, display, detect, make observable, and thereby accomplish an act's status as deviant" (1978, p. 280). While this position takes Becker's claims seriously, Scheff apparently never did. (Nor, for that matter, did Becker; see Pollner 1974, 1978.)

Scheff's version of labeling theory (1966) holds that *mental illness* is a classification people use to explain rule-breaking behavior when other culturally recognizable categories seem inappropriate. While ostensibly focusing on societal reaction as the essence of mental illness, the formulation is both conceptually flawed and carelessly applied to empirical cases. Scheff's use of the concept of residual rule breaking, for example, refers to the behavior of actors who are labeled rather than to the observers or reactors who apply the label. Hence, his focus remains on the putative deviant rather than on societal reaction. His application of labeling theory relies upon assertions about the qualities of acts that are defined by criteria other than responses to those acts. Mental illness, for Scheff, is *not* behavior so labeled. It is a distinctive kind of behavior—residual rule-breaking—that is subsequently labeled. The "deviant's" behavior—assessed by some "objective" standard—is the basis of the phenomenon "mental illness."

Of all the commentators on the Gove-Scheff debate, only Horwitz (1979) appears to have noticed Scheff's careless use of the labeling perspective. Remarking that Scheff was often unclear about whether mental illness refers to the behavior of the actor who displays "symptoms," or the process of ascription that assigns labels, Horwitz incisively noted that in Scheff's arguments, "Residual rule breaking, in fact, comes to be synonymous with the psychiatric concept of mental illness" (1979, p. 298). Not only is this a striking revelation (comparable, for example, to the discovery that "the emperor has no clothes"), but it also suggests that the adversaries in the labeling debate were fundamentally on the *same side* of the issue of just what mental illness is. Gove, for example, consistently argued that psychiatric symptoms distinguished involuntarily hospitalized mental patients from persons who were not committed. Scheff countered with claims that the contingencies of labeling were responsible for commitments; "social characteristics of the patients help determine the severity of the societal reaction, *independent of psychiatric condition*" (1974, p. 449, emphasis added). Note how this explicitly acknowledges an objectively ascertainable psychiatric condition as a phenomenon or condition independent of any constitutive labeling of it.

The admission that mental illness involves a form of symptomatic behavior is clear in Scheff's repeated insistence on "controlling" for psychiatric condition in empirical studies. In reviewing Haney and Michielutte's (1968) study of judicial determinations of incompetency, for example, Scheff states that they provide "only weak support [for labeling theory] since [they have] not controlled for the patient's condition" (1974, pp. 448–49). But Greenley's (1972) study, Scheff notes, found that "even when the patient's psychiatric condition is controlled, there is a strong relationship between family desire for the patient's release and the length of hospitalization" (1974, p. 449). By trying to ascertain and control for psychiatric condition, these studies treated mental condition as if it were objectively observable and assessable, abandoning any commitment to the radical labeling perspective.

Some of the studies Scheff cites to support the labeling perspective go to great lengths to provide psychiatric assessments that are independent of those rendered by the psychiatric personnel being studied. Wilde (1968), for example, examined protocols of psychiatric interviews with candidates for involuntary commitment to determine the extent to which these persons exhibited characteristics of committable mental illness. Wenger and Fletcher (1969) observed candidate patients during commitment hearings to determine if the psychiatric criteria for commitment were actually met. And Scheff (1964) himself observed judicial hearings to determine whether prospective patients were mentally ill according to legal criteria. When the observers in these studies found that candidate patients did not appear to be disturbed enough to warrant commitment, societal reaction to "social characteristics" was assigned responsibility for hearing outcomes.

Scheff's interest in controlling for mental illness or psychiatric condition suggests that his project was not to challenge the psychiatric model of mental illness, but rather to show that the model was poorly applied. The problem he locates in psychiatric labeling does not derive from the psychiatric model's conceptualization of mental illness; rather, it stems from errors in psychiatric decision-making. To demonstrate psychiatric errors, Scheff adopted the very concept of mental illness that he ostensibly attempted to displace. By attempting to show that psychiatric labels were often unwarranted, Scheff, and those he approvingly cites, acknowledged the possibility that some persons really were mentally ill and deserved to be labeled. In their studies, sociologist/observers assumed diagnostic authority and assessed the accuracy of psychiatric judgment. Faulting the psychiatric community, they implicitly suggested that detached observers were better judges of mental illness than were psychiatrists. The irony of this argument, however, lies in its thorough betrayal of the most distinctive and insightful claim of the labeling perspective—that mental illness was purely a social ascription. Instead of reconceptualizing mental illness, Scheff's version of labeling theory merely criticized psychiatric practice *in psychiatry's own terms*, thus helping to legitimize the psychiatric perspective at the same time he attacked its practice.

Constitutive Analysis

Conceding the conceptual debate over mental illness by default, labeling analysts could do little more than argue over the accuracy of psychiatric assessments. And as Horwitz (1979) noted, the debate made little headway toward fresh theoretical understandings. An analysis of constitutive interpretive practices, however, offers new perspective on mental illness and related issues. Most notably, it refuses to argue or compete with psychiatrists, judges, attorneys, or other practical actors regarding proper diagnoses, categorizations, or legal decisions. Instead, it reframes mental illness and the commitment process in terms of the processes through which reality is interpreted and represented, and attempts to describe the ways that persons involved in commitment proceedings produce and manage the realities that are implicated in commitment proceedings.

Most research on involuntary commitment has assumed that the "facts" that bear upon commitment proceedings correspond to features of an objectively knowable world. Decision-making is then conceptualized in terms of contingent relations between concrete variables. Studies have asked a range of questions like the following: Are the facts accurately known and adequately presented? What factors affect what is known and how it is presented? Is psychiatric condition more important in determining commitment decisions than nonpsychiatric factors? Are candidate patients' sex, age, race, or social class more influential than their psychiatric symptoms in predicting the outcomes of commitment proceedings? Does legal representation for the prospective patient or family preference regarding hospitalization or release affect the likelihood of commitment? Each question presupposes that an objective definition of each fact or variable is possible, and that the value of each variable can be assessed for each case. Commitment proceedings have employed externally imposed categories to capture the essence of what is going on as participants accomplish commitment decisions.

Imposing categories allows the classification and correlation of "second order constructs" (Schutz 1970), but it also reifies the phenomena as they are constructed by "outsiders," imposing decontextualized meanings without regard for how those develop within the situations being examined. Such an approach makes it possible to compare the ways members of situations act, react, and interact to externally developed models of rational action. Consequently, it encourages invidious critiques of members' practices, while failing to adequately explain, understand, or appreciate the indigenous or practical rationalities of everyday activity that members themselves fashion as they conduct their daily affairs.

Constitutive analysis, however, investigates and describes the things, actions, and meanings that actors within a social domain recognize and find intelligible. The focus is on methods of commonsense reasoning, criteria of choice, and practical means of evaluation as they are applied in everyday circumstances. Intersubjective knowledge, native understandings, and interpretive procedures are topical. Constitutive analysis of involuntary commitment proceedings thus centers on the interactional production and organization of the commitment process. Its interest in mental illness, psychiatric symptoms, or candidate patients' sex, age, or station in life is formulated in terms of how participants in the proceedings formulate and use these constructs to categorize and describe features of their experience and make sense of the circumstances they encounter.

The approach may superficially resemble Becker's or Scheff's labeling theories, but it rejects the "mundane" (Pollner 1974, 1978) understanding that "objective" characteristics, not the labeling process itself, constitute the phenomenon. In the mundane version, the deviant and nondeviant, the rule breaker and conformist, the rule-violating or compliant character of an act, are defined by some criterion other than the reactions of the community [e.g., residual rule breaking or psychiatric condition in Scheff's formulation, or obedient or rule-breaking behavior in Becker's (1963) version]. The application of labels then confers social judgment on the acts. As Pollner notes in describing the mundane approach:

> The community is conceived as an umpire whose task is to call balls and strikes. The relevant questions about the community's judgment focus on the extent to which they correspond to the act's "real" properties and the conditions affecting the correspondence. (1978:271)

A constitutive analysis, however, conceives community reaction as the sole source of deviant (or any) status, insisting that "deviance consists entirely and exclusively of the activities through which it is realized as such" (Pollner 1978, p. 279). There is "absolutely nothing else to consider other than the praxis through which persons orient to, display, detect, make observable, and thereby accomplish an act's status as deviant" (1978, p. 280). The deviance process no longer refers to those "intervening processes" through which deviance ascriptions are "correctly" or "incorrectly" attached, but rather is concerned with the practice through which deviants are constituted as recognizable entities in the first place. Constitutively, reaction refers to the entire method of responding to an act—perception, interpretation, representation, and evaluation. While mundane labeling theory is little more than a commonsense version of how social actors differentially respond to objectively deviant acts or phenomena, the constitutive version refocuses analytic attention on reality-creating processes.[1]

Taking a constitutive approach to involuntary commitment, this book analyzes how participants in commitment proceedings use their commonsense knowledge to produce reasoned and reasonable commitment decisions. Rather than attempting a "sociology of error" (Bloor 1976), trying to find fault with participants' practical reasoning, it describes the ways participants use descriptive categories, psychiatric constructs, and local knowledge of social roles and institutions to make accountable arguments for and against commitment. There is no need to determine the "real" mental status of candidates for commitment because the focus is on what commitment participants interpret to be real—mental illness as it is practically constituted.

Studying Interpretive Practice

The book, then, is about interpretive practice and involuntary commitment. Recalling Foucault, it examines the constitutive actions that divide *madness* from what is not considered *mad*. Foucault, however, provides a note of caution:

> It would certainly be a mistake to try to discover what could have been said of madness at a particular time by interrogating the being of madness itself, its secret content, its silent, self-enclosed truth; mental illness was constituted by all that was said in all the statements that named it, divided it up, described it, explained it, traced its developments, indicated its various correlations, judged it, and possibly gave it speech by articulating, in its name, discourses that were to be taken as its own. (1972, p. 32)

Accordingly, the book eschews a psychiatric or social scientific specification of the concept of mental illness in favor of analyzing everyday interactants' indigenous usage. To do otherwise would be to impose meaning that is external to the circumstances we are trying to understand. As Derrida (translated in Felman 1985) has remarked about Foucault's discussions of madness, any articulation or translation of madness gives it a particular form and meaning that derives from its situated and socially organized use—not from any essential character. Making everyday usage—the discourses of psychiatry, law, and commonsense reason—a topic for analysis allows us to circumvent the problem Derrida notes by analyzing acts of articulation that constitute practical realities.

Interpretive practice is reality-constructing activity—work that produces, manages, and sustains meaning. Commitment decision-making might therefore be called a form of "deviance or social problems work" (Miller and Holstein 1989). At the same time, considerable "normalizing work" goes on as part of typical commitment proceedings. The categories of *normal, sane, competent*, and the like, are interpretive resources just like their *deviance* counterparts.

Several themes characterize the discussion of interpretive practice. First, it is *interactional*. Consequently, the book examines language-mediated social interaction, focusing on how accountable decisions are interactionally accomplished. Second, the work is *political;* reality production and management is partisan activity, typically pitting one party's version against another's. Because alternative versions of reality compete, interpretive activity is *persuasive* and *rhetorical*. Finally, the interpretive work that constitutes commitment proceedings is *socially organized* and *organizational* in several senses. Interpretive practice organizes our understanding of actions, objects and circumstances, but these practices are themselves conditioned by circumstance. Consequently, interpretation and social structure stand in a reflexive relation, each providing the basis for the other. The book considers how the circumstances of commitment proceedings condition interpretive practice, providing the organized and organizational contexts and contingencies that influence interpretive work. It highlights locally preferred ways of understanding and talking, showing how descriptive practice is organizationally embedded—that is, conducted in concrete circumstances that provide parameters, discourses, and procedures to which members orient as they fashion commitment decisions.

Context and interpretive culture provide commonsense resources for depicting and understanding everyday experience, but interpretive practices must articulate available interpretive categories and schemas with the concrete circumstances at hand. Practical interpretation thus brings culturally understood images of madness and sanity, as well as images and discourses of other social forms (e.g., home and family), to bear on concrete cases where involuntary commitment is contemplated.

In a sense, then, the book is about how culture is articulated and enacted in the course of practical decision-making. It analyzes the ways that we discern and characterize the "normal" forms of everyday experience, as well as the "disturbed," "incompetent," and "deviant." Instance of mental disturbance and interactional incompetence, the book argues, are possible only by way of comparison with contrasting forms. Conversely, in looking at the features and circumstances of those who are involuntarily committed, we also glimpse the ways that contemporary society acknowledges its proper workings.

Note

1.   See Pollner (1974, 1978, and 1987) for further discussion of the distinction between the mundane version of labeling theory and its constitutive alternative. While most labeling studies have been in the mundane tradition, some have emphasized labeling's constitutive aspects without invoking distinctions between real and labeled deviance. See, for example, Emerson and Messinger (1977) or Kitsuse (1962, 1980).

Chapter 2

Analyzing Involuntary Commitment

If mental illness is a definitional or interpretive category that has come into conventional usage only relatively recently, attempting to trace the historical roots of the treatment of the mentally ill beyond those periods where the category has been available would be theoretically implausible. While Foucault and others offer histories of how societies have reacted differently to "madness" in various historical eras, the very essence of the interpretive argument is that the phenomenon itself is as varied as its interpretations. Madness was not somehow constant across eras, with only its labels and reactions varying. Rather, the diverse labels applied from era to era *constituted* distinctive sociohistorically located phenomena that cannot be treated as alternate representations of the same underlying reality.

A History of Involuntary Commitment

An attempt to outline a history of involuntary commitment must focus on how enforced confinement has been associated with the treatment of conditions known as mental illness. Historically, the labels *mad, insane,* and similar terms have often been used to segregate members from the general community. Most communities handled matters informally. Persons labeled *insane* were often warned off, sold at auction, confined to blockhouses or almshouses, or rounded up and deposited in other communities (Bell 1980). In the United States, however, some jurisdictions, enacted legislation permitting the detention of "mentally disturbed" persons under a variety of circumstances. Consider, for example, the mandate for controlling or confining persons in colonial Massachusetts:

"Whereas, There are distracted persons in some tounes, that are unruly, whereby not only the familyes wherein they are, but others suffer much damage by them, it is ordered by this court and the authoritye thereof, that the selectmen in all tounes where such persons are are hereby impowred & injoyned to take care of all such persons, that they doe not damnify others." (cited in Deutsch 1949, p. 43)

This order reveals two persistent and sometimes conflicting themes relating to mental disturbance. There is a clear concern for the "damage" that "distracted persons" might inflict on the community; the order explicitly instructs communities to protect members from such threats. But communities are also ordered to "take care of all such persons," suggesting a paternalistic responsibility to care for those who cannot fend for themselves. The order thus adumbrates the doctrine of *parens patriae* that has been at the heart of the debate regarding what to do about persons with mental deficiencies since the Progressive era.

During American colonial times, persons labeled insane, deranged, mad, and other related terms came to be regarded more sympathetically than in preceding eras. Following the lead of English reformer William Tuke and French physician Philippe Pinel, those concerned with the humane care of the insane advocated "moral treatment" as the progressive response. Exclusion and confinement were still the order of the day (Foucault 1965, 1987), but scientific, medical, and moral arguments began to insinuate the contemporary discourse about madness and its treatment. Pinel, for example, argued that mental stability was dependent upon a "balance of passions" and environmental stability; disorders were the result of excessive sentiments or desires (e.g., lust) or environmental disruptions (e.g., too much freedom or economic uncertainty). Pinel's recommendation was a program of reeducation through which persons were taught how to behave normally within the context of sympathetic living conditions (Cockerham 1981).[1]

Responses to those labeled insane, however, were not compelled in any straightforward fashion by developing moral, medical, or psychiatric doctrines or discoveries. Mental health treatment did not progressively "evolve" from its unsophisticated predecessors. Rather, responses to madness often involved a variety of techniques, sometimes mixing moral teaching with social precaution and medical strategy (Foucault 1965, 1987). In this climate, early attempts at institutional treatment began to develop. "Lunaticks," for example, were admitted to the Pennsylvania Hospital beginning in 1752 (Appelbaum and Kemp 1982), and mental asylums were founded in the early eighteenth century. Benjamin Rush, the "father" of American psychiatry, introduced "moral treatment" to the Pennsylvania Hospital around the turn of the nineteenth century, while institutions such as the Worcester (Massachusetts)

State Hospital were held as examples of enlightenment for the rest of the country (Cockerham 1981; Gallagher 1987).

With a version of psychiatric treatment and mental hospitalization now available, concern shifted to ways of assuring service to persons thought to be in need of treatment. Deutsch (1949) suggests that individuals considered mentally disordered were progressively more likely to be institutionalized through the late eighteenth and early nineteenth centuries. The authority to confine disturbed persons remained more or less informal. Family members and physicians could institute confinement for treatment without regard for the patient's rights or wishes. In Pennsylvania, for example, hospitals allowed mentally disturbed persons to be admitted, regardless of the persons' desires, on the petition of a family member or friend. The petition was to be accompanied by a physician's certification of the patient's "insanity." Deutsch illustrated the ease and informality with which treatment could be imposed by noting that Benjamin Rush had admitted a patient by merely scrawling "James Sproul [the patient] is a proper patient for the Pennsylvania Hospital" on a scrap of paper (1949, p. 442). Hospitals were typically more concerned about the ability of patients or their friends or relatives to pay for hospitalization than they were about depriving patients of their freedom, or enforcing treatment without the patients' consent.

Legal challenges to involuntary confinement were rare during the early nineteenth century. Indeed, there were few safeguards, while family members had extensive power to commit allegedly disturbed persons. For example, in 1849 Morgan Hinchman, an escapee from the Friend's Asylum in Pennsylvania, brought suit against his family and friends for conspiring to commit him to the facility in order to gain control of his property. Both sides agreed that Hinchman had been forcibly detained in the asylum, and that considerable property was subsequently confiscated. They disagreed, however, about Hinchman's mental condition. The defendants argued that Hinchman had exhibited symptoms—some of them violent—for years, and had been squandering his assets, including his wife's inheritance. Hinchman, however, produced several local witnesses who swore that Hinchman was, in fact, sane.

The judge in the cases instructed the jury that if Hinchman had been insane at the time of his commitment, his friends and family could not be held liable for conspiring to deprive him of his rights because they had intended to act in his best interest by hospitalizing him. The judge thus held that no legal process was required to commit the truly insane:

"If confinement or restraint, with regular medical treatment, are necessary for the restoration of such a person to a perfectly sound state of mind, they

are the best friends of the party who enforce it." (cited in Appelbaum and
Kemp 1982, p. 347)

Although some of the defendants were found guilty of conspiracy, the
common-law right of family and friends to restrain the nondangerous
insane for their own benefit was reaffirmed; informal commitment could
continue (Appelbaum and Kemp 1982).

Most accounts of the development of commitment laws describe a
rather abrupt midcentury shift away from liberal criteria honoring family
prerogatives and physicians' medical discretion (Appelbaum and Kemp
1982). The conflict between concerns for paternalism and autonomy began to come into sharper focus as activists began to campaign both for
more and better facilities for treating the mentally disturbed and for
judicial protection from involuntary treatment. Dorothea Dix, for example, was appalled at the conditions facing disturbed persons living in the
community. With the popular press helping to publicize the deplorable
conditions faced by the insane, she launched national and international
campaigns to construct new mental hospitals. Her aim, however, was
mainly to improve treatment, and she was far less concerned about the
legal rights of prospective patients (Rothman 1971).

At about the same time, Mrs. E. P. W. Packard became the focus of a
controversial effort to secure judicial safeguards against the deprivation
of liberty in the name of involuntary treatment. Mrs. Packard had apparently disagreed with her husband regarding religious beliefs, and in
1860 he had her confined and treated for mental disturbance in an Illinois hospital. Mrs. Packard objected, but under existing state law, her
husband's recommendation in conjunction with the approval of the
medical superintendent was sufficient to hospitalize her. Upon her release, Mrs. Packard began a campaign to require judicial oversight, and
Illinois subsequently instituted mandatory jury trials for involuntary
commitment, while other states apparently followed suit (Bell 1980).

Whereas the generally accepted version of the development of commitment laws argues that judicial safeguards for the process emerged
rather quickly, Appelbaum and Kemp (1982) argue that changes were
not so precipitous, nor were they immediately widespread. They cite the
evolution of commitment procedures in Pennsylvania as an example.
With the opening of Pennsylvania's first state hospital for the insane at
Harrisburg in 1851, two mechanisms for civil commitment were for-
malized. A court could commit an individual whose insanity was established in the manner provided by law and who was "unsafe to be at
large," or who was "suffering any unnecessary duress or hardship."
Alternatively, the administrators of the poor laws could commit "insane

paupers under their charge as they may deem proper subjects" (Appelbaum and Kemp 1982, p. 346).

While the first provision seemed to represent a move toward judicial control, the statute was not motivated by desire for formal procedures. The state hospital's bylaws continued to permit the admission of patients on the request of family members when accompanied by a physician's certification of insanity if the patients' hospitalization would be paid for. The new statute may thus have represented merely an attempt to establish a means to define those patients for whom the state would pay—that is, those who were not cared for by family or friends or who were dangerous or disruptive of the public order (Appelbaum and Kemp 1982). The law clearly supported family members' and public administrators' rights to act without judicial oversight.

By the late 1860s, however, the courts' attitude toward informal commitment began to change. A series of cases heard by Judge Brewster provided the occasion for the judiciary to articulate a newfound concern for the deprivation of liberty. Brewster handed down a set of rulings that all but invalidated informal commitment procedures, seemingly creating a system of exclusive judicial commitment. In response to Richard Nye's writ of habeas corpus demanding his release from the Pennsylvania Hospital, Brewster concluded that it was wrong for a man's liberty to depend upon decisions made by his physician and family, let alone a single judge. He ruled that without a formal "finding of lunacy" by a jury, not even a judge could commit a patient to "imprisonment for life" (Appelbaum and Kemp 1982, p. 347).

In a subsequent case, Brewster invalidated a physician's finding of lunacy that was based totally on the testimony of the patient's sons, who had initiated both commitment proceedings and criminal charges. " 'If such proceedings [which did not include an examination of the patient by the physician] can be tolerated,' Brewster argued, 'our constitution and laws, professing to guard human liberty, are all wastepaper' " (cited in Appelbaum and Kemp 1982, p. 348). And, in yet another commitment case, Brewster ruled that even a lunacy hearing was insufficient basis for commitment. He concluded that commitment was invalid without a court order, thereby abandoning the common-law assumption that family and friends would act in the best interest of a patient.

The traditional interpretation of the history of psychiatric hospitalization suggests that judicial oversight progressively supplanted family and physician discretion for the remainder of the century. Appelbaum and Kemp (1982), however, point out that in the wake of the Brewster rulings, the Pennsylvania legislature debated alternative commitment statutes and finally adopted a bill that upheld informal commitment for persons with responsible friends or family. Judicial commitment was permitted when a court was notified of an individual's insanity and need for hospitalization, and judges were given discretion to order commitment for insane persons in need of care or treatment. The Pennsylvania legislature thus overturned the judicial decisions that prohibited informal commitment at precisely the time that judicial control seemed to be ascending.

While public debate continued about the need for judicial supervision, both in Pennsylvania, and across the nation, it appears that conflicting arguments prevailed at different times and places. Those interested in the need for treatment, the protection of the community, procedural guarantees, and the preservation of individual rights and liberty all won important victories regarding the detention and treatment of the insane. So, while judicial control over involuntary commitment was certainly more prominent than at the outset of the century, it was something short of predominant or consistent by 1900. Indeed, a curious patchwork of schemes for involuntary commitment had emerged by this time: Five states permitted hospitalization by order of a justice of the peace, eighteen permitted only judges to confine mental patients, five required lay jury trials, three required juries that included at least one physician, three used court-appointed commissions, two used asylum boards, and nine required only medical certification. Although dangerousness was sometimes a criterion for commitment, there is no indication that hospitalization was generally limited to persons considered dangerous (Shuman 1985).

Gradually, over the next fifty years, advances in medicine and psychiatry bolstered arguments that the mentally ill should be hospitalized for therapeutic reasons, eroding many of the earlier legal protections (Levenson 1986; Shuman 1985). Rigid procedures resembling criminal proceedings were regarded as antitherapeutic measures that frustrated treatment efforts and traumatized helpless patients. By the late 1940s, mental health professionals were arguing that procedural safeguards were outdated—that they were a response to circumstances that had ceased to exist. Modern mental institutions and improved psychiatric treatments, they argued, mitigated prior concerns for the welfare of persons confined for treatment.

The 1960s, however, witnessed a growing reaction to the relaxed attitude. A number of judicial decisions—mainly involving criminal matters—called into question the notion that psychiatric advances and benevolent intentions were an adequate substitute for judicial safeguards. Confinement, whether designed as punishment or treatment, was progressively viewed as a deprivation of liberty requiring due process. The shift in attitude generalized to the mentally ill. By the 1970s, a

series of judicial decisions had begun to support the constitutional necessities of notifying candidate patients of their rights, allowing them to
be present at commitment hearings, providing them with adequate legal
counsel, and other procedural safeguards that had practically disappeared (Shuman 1985).

Contemporary Involuntary Commitment Laws

In the 1960s and 1970s, a wave of reformed involuntary commitment
legislation was enacted across the United States, providing candidates
for involuntary commitment with many—if not all—due process rights
accorded defendants in criminal proceedings. While there has been yet
another round of reforms and proposals for relaxation of procedural
safeguards in recent years (see Wexler 1988), the involuntary commitment statutes discussed in this book were influenced by, if not modeled
after California's Lanterman-Petris-Short Act (LPS), which went into
effect in 1969 and was modified in 1974.

Like most reformed involuntary commitment legislation, LPS tried to
balance individuals' due process rights against needs to help and protect
persons who are incapable of serving their own best interests, and concerns for safeguarding the community from dangerous or disruptive
members. Briefly, the legislation provides for a variety of options for
involuntary evaluation and commitment. All commitments begin with a
seventy-two-hour hold period for evaluation and treatment in a psychiatric facility. The hold requires the certification of a physician who is a
staff member at the designated treatment facility, a peace officer, or other
designated "mental health" personnel. The candidate patient must be
certified as both mentally disordered and either a danger to him- or
herself, a danger to others, or "gravely disabled"—that is, unable to
provide food, clothing, and/or shelter—as a result of the disorder.

By the end of the seventy-two-hour detention, a psychiatrist must
determine whether to release the patient or to secure the patient's
commitment—either voluntarily or involuntarily. The next phase of involuntary commitment involves a fourteen-day certification for observation and treatment. When this expires, persons deemed dangerous
to self—those considered to be imminently suicidal—may be detained
for an additional fourteen days. They must, however, be released at the
end of this second period, even if they are still considered suicidal. Persons considered dangerous to others must be released after the initial
fourteen-day commitment, or be recommitted for ninety days (with the
possibility of renewing the order). Formal judicial hearings are mandatory for all ninety-day commitments.[2]

Technically, then, the state may detain persons for evaluation and treatment without formal "commitment hearings." But persons committed involuntarily may file writs of habeas corpus to seek judicial review and release at any time during either the fourteen-day or ninety-day certifications. Most of the proceedings observed for this book were of this type and will be called *commitment hearings* throughout. Persons whose commitment was under consideration were already mental patients, if only temporarily. While I refer to them as *patients*, this does not necessarily endorse the status assignment.

LPS also provides for patients' due process rights, although such rights are not as vigorously protected as those of criminal defendants. Patients have the right to be present at all hearings, and must be notified in advance of the time and place of all proceedings in which they are involved. They have the right to competent legal counsel, and court-appointed representation will be provided if patients are unable to secure the services of a private attorney. Patients, however, may not be accompanied by counsel during psychiatric interviews.

The burden of proof in habeas corpus hearings and other commitment proceedings lies with the state, which must establish that the patient is both mentally disordered and meets at least one of the three criteria for commitment under LPS. The constitutional standard for commitment is "clear and convincing evidence." Evidence must be produced through direct testimony, although hearsay evidence from a patient's psychiatric record is frequently introduced without challenge. Records from any past medical treatment may be introduced.

Commitment laws across the United States—including four of the jurisdictions observed for this study—are generally similar to those in California. The most common difference lies in the technical requirements and guidelines for initial commitment hearings. Most jurisdictions typically specify mandatory judicial review soon after the initial commitment. Sometimes the review takes the form of a preliminary hearing to determine if probable cause for detention exists, and if a formal commitment hearing should be scheduled. While a preliminary hearing was necessary to initiate any involuntary detention in one of the jurisdictions studied, more typically the initial hearing takes place three to five days after the patient is first detained. Formal hearing sometimes take place seventeen days or more after the initiation of commitment actions.

Criteria for involuntary commitment in other jurisdictions generally resemble California's. Evidence of mental disorder is required, and danger to self and/or others is statutorily defined as grounds for involuntary hospitalization. Definitions and specifications of danger vary, and sometimes require evidence of a recent overt act (or pattern of acts) that suggests a substantial probability of injury to self or others. Alternatively, some statutes specify that commitment is warranted if a mentally disturbed person's judgment is "sufficiently impaired" that he or she is likely to bring harm to him- or herself.

Many jurisdictions vary regarding what California calls grave disability. Several employ California's term and definition, while others explicitly stipulate that the inability to meet basic needs for food, clothing, shelter, medical care, and personal safety are aspects of danger to self. By failing to provide food, clothing, shelter, and so forth, it is argued, a mentally disordered person is endangering his or her own well-being, and is therefore dangerous to him- or herself.

Research Settings

The data analyzed here come from several settings where involuntary commitments were considered. The most important of these were involuntary commitment hearings themselves, although I also observed informal discussions in other settings where commitment matters were informally negotiated—the halls and waiting areas of a courthouse, for example. Intermittently, from 1981 through 1990, I observed commitment proceedings and related activities in five jurisdictions across the United States. I supplemented my observations with formal and informal interviews with participants in the commitment process, including judges, attorneys representing the state, persons whose commitment was under consideration and their attorneys, psychiatrists, psychologists, social workers, and other mental health professionals.

Metropolitan Court

Most of my fieldwork was conducted in Metropolitan Court in California from 1981 through 1984.[3] This court serves a large, cosmopolitan urban area and hears only cases related to mental health issues. Proceedings are governed by LPS. During the course of my observations, two judges presided over the vast majority of the habeas corpus cases, although several others appeared as substitutes during vacations and other absences by the regular judges. All the judges were male, and all but one short-term substitute were white. Occasionally, Metropolitan Court judges would be asked to preside over jury trials involving mental health–related issues, but their primary task is to rule on habeas corpus writs.

At any one time there were three to six representatives of the district attorney's (DA) office working at Metropolitan Court. Their role is to argue the state's case that patients should be confined for the period for which they had been certified. In many respects, they served as prosecutors in the proceedings. A similar number of representatives of the public defender's (PD) office provided counsel for most of the patients who sought their release in court. Only very rarely was a patient represented by a private attorney. The court attorneys formed a racially and sexually diverse group. The DAs and PDs all carried large caseloads, each typically having several hearings scheduled each day. Case records were routinely reviewed before court went into session, but it was not uncommon for the attorneys to meet and interview patients only on the morning of their scheduled hearing. Many of these interviews were conducted in the hallways and waiting room outside the courtroom, with court personnel scrambling to match persons with records before their cases were called.

Each year, about three thousand persons file writs in Metropolitan Court. This population is racially and ethnically diverse, reflecting the heterogeneity of the metropolitan area; about half of the petitioners are white (Anglo), while the remainder are African American, Hispanic, Asian, and Middle Eastern. About 60 percent of the cases I observed involved male patients and about 60 percent involved persons between the ages of twenty and forty. Most patients appeared to be of relatively low socioeconomic status.

Patients come to Metropolitan Court from psychiatric facilities around the metropolitan area. These include a large state psychiatric hospital, VA hospitals, and a variety of other public and private facilities. Court sessions usually began at 10:00 A.M. with the daily calendar call, and continued until late afternoon. Patients arrived in buses, vans, and other smaller vehicles, and were usually loosely supervised by psychiatric personnel from the holding facilities. Sometimes their supervisors were the psychiatrists or psychologists who were also going to testify against them in court. More commonly, "psych techs" and other custodians from the hospitals were responsible for keeping track of the patients while they waited for their hearings to begin, and while they marked time until they would return to their respective psychiatric facilities.

Metropolitan Court is located in a large brick building in a neighborhood consisting of industrial, commercial, and residential developments, directly across the street from frequently traveled railroad tracks. The building houses two large courtrooms (one used for habeas corpus hearings, the other for conservatorship hearings), administrative offices, and a large, starkly furnished "waiting" area. Petitioners typically wandered around or sat on benches in the waiting area and open hallways, or in the courtroom gallery awaiting their appearance in court.

A stranger to the courthouse might find the setting somewhat surreal.

Patients—all current residents of psychiatric wards—moved freely about the premises, walking, sitting, chatting with others, even speaking to no one in particular. Some displayed what insiders recognize as side effects of psychotropic medications—drooling, involuntary muscular contractions, and the inability to remain still for even the shortest interval. Others were openly "delusional," speaking of things that most persons would consider bizarre if not impossible. On any particular day, an observer might hear someone claim to be a past president of the United States, a movie star, an alien from outer space, or Jesus Christ. But the same observer would also hear numerous conversations no more peculiar than those heard in any public meeting place, for example, cafeterias, bus stops, grocery stores, or baseball games.

Patients arrived in various states of attire, ranging from the sort of dress clothing typically expected for courtroom appearances, to neat casual attire, to piecemeal, disheveled outfits, to institutionally issued pajamas. Interspersed were a variety of "appropriately dressed" courtroom personnel and observers. Mental patients, office workers, lawyers, psychiatrists, MDs, social service workers, and students from two local universities were regulars at Metropolitan Court. Patients intermingled freely, so it was often difficult, if not impossible, to determine casually who was who. I used the following rule of thumb for making quick assessments: Persons carrying briefcases were typically attorneys, those with clipboards or file folders were psychiatrists, those with badges of various sorts were peace officers or psych techs, and those gathered together, looking on apprehensively, were apt to be students or observers. Others could be court employees, persons having business in the court building, or habeas corpus petitioners.

For the most part, I conducted my observations as unobtrusively as possible. I sat or stood in the halls and waiting areas, and viewed the court proceedings from the gallery, usually to one side or the other, near the front. Over time, the court regulars (judges, attorneys, psych techs, and even some oft-returning petitioners) began to recognize me, although I was often mistaken for a court worker, occasionally a psychiatrist, or more frequently a patient. When asked about my presence, I easily explained myself as a sociologist interested in how commitment hearings were conducted.

There are a variety of perspectives from which to view the proceedings in Metropolitan Court. I chose to be unobtrusive hoping to view the scene without obstruction, while minimally altering it with my presence. My interest was primarily in the courtroom interactions, and except for being barred from tape-recording the proceedings, I had complete access to this aspect of the proceedings. I also did numerous informal interviews with the participants in the commitment process when the opportunity spontaneously arose. I often approached attorneys, psychiatrists, judges, and petitioners with questions about the court's activities, their perspectives on some activity I had observed, or simply their general impressions of the commitment process. Some of these became extended interviews, while others were casual chats between other more pressing duties in their daily rounds. Much of the dead time around the courthouse (e.g., before court went into session, between sessions, or at lunch breaks) was spent talking casually with patients, their attendants, and occasionally other courtroom personnel who had a free moment.

There are advantages and disadvantages to the various locations within the "field" from which one might choose to observe. Carol Warren (1982), for example, has also done extensive observation in Metropolitan Court, but her studies were conducted from a substantially different perspective. Whereas I chose the stance of an unobtrusive outsider, Warren gained access to the court through the judge and viewed proceedings from a desk directly beside his dais. She had full access to court documents, off-the-record conversations, and other sorts of information and experience not as easily available to me. In particular, her studies reveal details of considerable backstage activity, of which I was only vaguely aware and to which I had only sporadic access. But her special status in the court also had its disadvantages, most notably the assumption by other courtroom personnel that she was the "judge's own person" (see Warren 1982, pp. 215–39). Since I had the advantage of Warren's published insights into the court's backstage activities, and was most interested in the dynamics of commitment hearings themselves, I felt less need to explore those areas opened to her because of her privileged status. Instead, I focused my observations on the public proceedings and tried to capture them as naturalistically as possible. Thus, Warren and I frequently offer contrasting portraits of the court. But they do not represent conflicting assessments of what was going on as much as they formulate different aspects of the phenomenon as viewed from different physical, interpretive, and theoretical perspectives. I believe our work is largely complementary, and recommend her studies to anyone interested in the involuntary commitment process, or the sociology of mental illness more generally.

Other Study Sites

The vast majority of my observations were done in Metropolitan Court, but I also studied the commitment process on a more limited basis in four other jurisdictions. I observed at least one commitment hearing in each of these locales, and conducted interviews with judges,[4] patients, psychiatric and social service workers, law enforcement personnel, and others who might have been involved in the commitment process. "Eastern Court" was located in a medium-sized city (approximate population two hundred thousand) near the geographic center of a large eastern state. "Southern Court" served several counties of a southeastern state, including one medium-sized city (population approximately three hundred thousand) and extensive rural areas. "Midland Court" was located in a metropolitan area with a population of well over one million in the upper Midwest. And "Northern Court" served an isolated, sparsely populated (approximately twenty thousand) rural county in the northern Midwest.[5]

Legislation governing commitment proceedings is generally similar in all of these jurisdictions and resembles California's LPS. One notable exception is that none of these explicitly use the term *grave disability* as a criterion for involuntary mental hospitalization. One state explicitly defines dangerousness to self as the "inability to meet basic needs of food, shelter, medical care or safety such that without prompt and adequate treatment death, serious disability, physical injury, or serious physical disease will imminently ensue." The criterion thus effectively mirrors California's grave disability criterion. In the other jurisdictions, failure to provide for basic needs is also considered an endangerment to self, so all of the jurisdictions studied do commit persons based on de facto provisions for grave disability, or something very much like it.

Another difference in commitment statutes appears in the inclusion in three states of wording that stipulates that persons may be involuntarily committed if they are "in need of treatment." This directive may appear within definitions of either mental disorder or mental illness (e.g., mental disturbances to such an extent that the afflicted person requires care, treatment, and rehabilitation) in a somewhat tautological fashion, or in specifications of dangerousness criteria (e.g., dangerous so as to require confinement and treatment). While such statutes have become the focus for some legal controversy (see Mestrovic 1983), my observations suggest that despite statutory differences, similar legal and psychiatric concerns and orientations operate in all of the sites studied.

In all jurisdictions, the proceedings I call *commitment hearings* were held after an initial hospitalization for care and evaluation. The persons whose commitment was under consideration were technically patients at the time, so their hearings were like California's habeas corpus hearings in that regard.

Commitment Hearings in Brief

Involuntary commitment hearings are conducted very similarly in the five jurisdictions studied, following the format described in the Introduction. The state's attorney calls a psychiatrist to provide the psychiatric argument for commitment.[6] The attorney for the person whose commitment is under consideration then cross-examines. After this, the patient is called to testify as to why he or she should be released, and the state's attorney cross-examines. The judge then renders a decision. It is more likely that other witnesses will be called in the non-California sites, but most cases in all jurisdictions hear testimony from only the doctor and the patient.

While the law states that the *treating psychiatrist* must offer testimony regarding the patient's mental condition, this is often not the case in Metropolitan Court. Most of the persons filing writs were held in large local psychiatric facilities and several might have hearings in Metropolitan Court each day. If the law were to be strictly observed, each patient's treating psychiatrist would have to accompany the patient to court, and might spend the entire day waiting for the case to be called. Consequently, staff psychiatrists at the facilities typically agreed among themselves to testify in hearings involving patients for whom they were not the treating psychiatrists, thus limiting the number who had to go to court, and preserving the clinical schedules at their institutions.

The testifying doctors had access to patient records and may have been familiar with the patients, their diagnoses, and treatment histories and plans before the day of their court appearances. At minimum they would review the psychiatric records, and attempt to briefly interview the patient, often in the halls of the court building itself. The PD's office stipulated that the presence of treating psychiatrists could be waived in order to allow the psychiatric facilities to remain adequately staffed. Thus, the proceedings at Metropolitan Court might involve a single psychiatrist from the state hospital, for example, who would testify in the hearings of several patients—none of whom might actually be under his or her care.

Cases proceeded in a remarkably routine pattern, given some of the unusual claims that were heard. As Warren (1982) suggests, this is not because the proceedings are perfunctory or because participants view the court's work as inconsequential. Rather, a "working consensus" on the practices and interpretations that characterize everyday life in Metropolitan Court has been built up over the years, so that an attitude of "we all work together here" (Warren 1982, p. 140) discourages procedural squabbles and challenges, moves that might be legally reasonable but practically disruptive.

The bedrock of routine understandings is most evident in its absence, that is, at times when "outsiders" participated in habeas corpus writ hearings. Occasionally, due to judges' vacations or other professional obligations, or instances when private attorneys represented patients, or when psychiatrists attempted to make the case for commitment without the assistance of an attorney, strangers would occupy the familiar roles of the courtroom regulars. In these instances, violations of routine by the newcomers might result in a flurry of procedural objections that could transform the proceedings from smoothly run, rather informal adjudications into legal "nitpicking" that invariably undermined the "newcomer's" ability to function in the court and disrupted the proceedings considerably.[7]

Hearings in the other jurisdictions were basically similar. Psychiatrists and patients testified, they were cross-examined, and very infrequently a family member or social service worker might be called to testify. In all instances, the judges interacted freely with witnesses, asking questions as the cases proceeded. Northern Court and Eastern Court commitment hearings took place in standard courtrooms that were used for other cases as well. Judges in both jurisdictions routinely cleared the courtroom for commitment cases, although each admitted that such hearings were technically open to the public. The judges suggested that there was no need to gratuitously intrude upon patients' privacy, and each suggested that the trauma of court hearings should be minimized so as to not exacerbate the patients' psychiatric disturbances.

Citing the same rationale, the judge in Southern Court literally went to the patients to hold commitment hearings. In the company of a court clerk, the judge drove to the facility holding the patient and conducted the hearing on site. In one of the cases I observed, for example, the judge met with the patient in the library of a private psychiatric hospital. There, around a conference table, the judge, a representative of the state attorney's office, and an attorney paid by the county to represent the patient questioned the patient and the treating psychiatrist in much the same fashion as witnesses were questioned in Metropolitan Court. Finally, commitment cases in Midland are held in a special courtlike hearing room located in the County Mental Health Complex. The personnel and proceedings here were similar to those already described.

Hearing outcomes varied across the sites studied. According to the first judge in Metropolitan Court, about 60 percent of his cases resulted in hospitalization, although his commitment rate was slightly lower for the cases I observed. The other judges in Metropolitan Court reported that they had commitment rates somewhat higher than this. Indeed, one temporary judge never granted a writ releasing a patient. In the other jurisdictions, commitment hearings usually—but not always—resulted in hospitalization; judges' informal estimates of commitment rates ranged from 60 to 90 percent. Commitment decisions, then, are not foregone conclusions. While commitment is statistically more likely, release is not rare.

Methodological Approach

Commitment hearings offer an opportunity to observe interpretive practice regarding matters we typically take for granted and ignore in the course of everyday life—matters like identity, sanity, normalcy, and competence. Courts of any sort are particularly good sites for viewing the way actors describe, interpret, theorize about, and determine what is real. As Pollner (1987) suggests, they provide attractive opportunities for inspecting the practices of mundane reason through which the life world is constructed and sustained.

Whereas participants argue and conjecture about facts and outcomes, they nonetheless assume that the things they contest and dispute do, in fact, exist independently of the interpretive and judgmental acts in which they are engaged. Constitutive analysis, however, attempts to render these phenomena problematic by focusing on interaction that constructs what is "real." Commitment hearings provide a rich opportunity to examine how taken-for-granted features of our everyday lives, experiences, and identities are assembled through routinely "seen but unnoticed" (Garfinkel 1967) interactional practices.

The concern for reality-constituting practices is explicitly ethnomethodological (see Garfinkel 1967; Heritage 1984), focusing the study on how the organized and understandable features of commitment hearings and their participants are accomplished. The dynamics of interaction and the discourse are of central interest. Interpretation is not construed as a merely cognitive operation—something going on inside people's heads. Rather, it is public, interactional, and representational.

Framing interpretation and decision-making as fundamentally social focuses attention on how participants in commitment proceedings indicate, describe, and discursively orient to the relevant factors in commitment decision-making. Participants' talk is the phenomenon of interest. Social scientists have long-standing and well-documented concerns with how to analyze subjects' discourse. Conventional apprehensions include the fear that, at worst, subjects might lie to researchers. Nearly as disquieting is the suspicion that subjects might not reveal all they know, thus concealing the full truth from researchers. An even more daunting concern, however, is the fear of distorting or contaminating what subjects might have otherwise said by the mere act of making them the focus of research. This is the classic problem of "reactivity"—changing the phenomenon though acts of observation.

My research strategy was to be as unobtrusive as possible. I am confident that my presence in most of the scenes I describe was either not noticed or thoroughly ignored by the persons being observed. Of course there were instances—especially in closed hearings like those held by the Southern Court judge—where my presence was conspicuous. Because the proceedings I observed did not seem to vary according to the salience of my presence, I am reasonably confident that it minimally disrupted normal activities.

Analysis always depends on a theory of what subjects' discourse represents, even if the theory is implicit. Conventional social science typically rests on both a correspondence theory of meaning—that is, that the meaning of words lies in what they reference or stand for—and the notion that what people say should be consistent with what they do. This assumed relationship between talk and action, however, has proved elusive. Considerable social psychological research, for example, demonstrates that what people do and what they say they will do or say they have done, are not highly correlated (see Heritage 1983). This is not to say, however, that people are merely untruthful or inaccurate.

An alternative perspective on analyzing talk suggest that accounts and explanations are not "just talk" about some other state of affairs that might be more or less truthful. Rather, talk—descriptions, accounts, arguments, and explanation—may be analyzed as action in its own right (Heritage 1983; Mills 1940). Focusing on those problematic occasions when people are called upon to explain or justify their actions and decisions—circumstances not unlike commitment proceedings—Mills (1940) notes that explanations commonly take the form of normatively acceptable accounts, that is, accounts that would be heard by relevant others as reasonable and acceptable. They are formulated with the objective of appealing to an audience. In addition, the contours of what could pass for a satisfactory explanation are influenced by the social context or institutional circumstance in which accounts are rendered.

But accounts are not merely post hoc justifications for actions. Mills argued that actors anticipate the need for local, normative accountability, formulating behavior so as to provide for the possibility of employing the normative vocabulary of plausible accounts for the purpose of explanation. As Mills suggests, "Often anticipations of acceptable justifications will control conduct" (1940, p. 907). The relationship between talk and action, then, is complex, with the possibility that either one might motivate the other. This analysis is not concerned with how instances of talk represent cognitive decision-making, nor with the "real reasons" that may privately exist for persons' words and actions. Instead, it analyzes instances of talk during commitment proceedings as consequential acts in their own right. Arguments and explanations are treated as participants' ways of displaying the reasonableness, rationality, and legality of the business at hand.

That business transpires in particular institutional, organizational, historical, and cultural environments, making context consequential to interpretive practice. Analysis must therefore be sensitive to the ways that interaction and interpretation are conditioned or constrained by practical circumstance. The challenge is to discern and describe how situational contingencies and local cultures (Gubrium 1989, 1991)—that is, more or less regularized and localized possibilities for assigning meaning and responding to persons and things—are incorporated into interpretive practice.

These analytic concerns require a methodological approach focused on contextually grounded interaction and discourse. The procedures I have followed in collecting and analyzing data might best be characterized as "ethnography of practice" (Gubrium 1988) or "constitutive ethnography" (Mehan 1979). The approach appreciates both local enactment and contextual resources and orientations. My observations in and around involuntary commitment proceedings typically began with conventional ethnographic concerns for understanding "what was going on." The study began in Metropolitan Court, where I initially familiarized myself with the settings and participants, then tried to discern how the court and its activity were understood by its participants. This process generated a profusion of field notes, often unsystematically recorded and unfocused. Progressively, my note-taking became more focused and purposeful. Outside the courtroom I would talk with, and informally interview, many of the people who were involved in the commitment proceedings, asking questions that clarified my understanding of how they viewed the proceedings. Inside the courtroom, during the actual commitment hearings, I initially attempted to note the broader dynamics of the courtroom interaction and ritual. After several weeks, however, my concern for talk-in-interaction focused my note-taking more narrowly on courtroom conversation.

I would have videotaped commitment hearings if this were possible. No recordings were permitted, however, so I attempted to take detailed notes on exactly what was said, to the best of my ability. This is not a perfect substitute, but it was the best alternative under the circumstances.[8] By trying to take verbatim notes on conversation, I undoubtedly missed considerable nonverbal interaction that was taking place as I wrote. More importantly, the richness and accuracy of my data were severely compromised by my hearing and note-taking abilities. Indeed, there are several sources of "bias" embedded in my note-taking procedures. Segments of talk that were clearly enunciated and slowly paced were more easily captured. Formulaic or brief exchanges of questions and answers were easily noted, as was talk marked by repeated or extended silence. Conversely, rapid talk, extended continuous utterances, and poorly articulated testimony were difficult to note. On several occasions in Metropolitan Court, I was accompanied by students, colleagues, or friends. I usually asked them to record the talk of a single person involved in the proceedings. Combining these notes with my own often produced some of the more detailed transcriptions in my collection.

While my transcriptions fell considerably short of perfection—varying in quality from segment to segment, case to case—they proved to be good "field notes" in the sense that they captured the general sense of what was being said very well. But, as my analytic interest in the organization of hearing discourse led me to greater concerns with the specific details of conversational structure, the data became progressively less adequate because my near-transcriptions failed to capture all the fine-grained detail of actual conversation-in-progress. Nevertheless, my data collection procedures were my best effort to adapt to the practical circumstances constraining the study.

For most of the analysis that follows, my field data are sufficiently detailed to capture the general sense and flow of interaction during commitment hearings. In all, I observed and took notes on over four hundred habeas corpus writ hearings in Metropolitan Court (most of these from 1982 to 1984), and approximately twenty-nine other commitment hearings in the other field sites.

While I attempt close descriptions of conversational structure and dynamics in some parts of my analysis, I do not claim that they adhere to the technical standards of rigor applied in conventional conversation analysis (see Atkinson and Heritage 1984). Atkinson and Drew (1979) offer a rationale for the use of detailed field notes on conversational exchanges and "do-it-yourself" transcripts that I have also adopted: Do the best you can with the available materials and circumstances. Therefore, I have used my field notes as well as a collection of near-transcriptions to analyze courtroom discourse in as great detail as possible. The near-transcriptions note what was being said as well as several relevant features of the conversations, including the occurrence of silences, longer pauses, and simultaneous speech. In all, I have analyzed near-transcriptions of fifty-five extended segments of direct examination of patients by public defenders, sixty-seven extended segments of cross-examination of patients by representatives of the district attorney's office, seventy-one extended segments of psychiatrists' testimony, and approximately three hundred shorter segments of talk by the various participants in the hearings.

* * * * *

This book focuses on the discourse in and around commitment hearings, describing and analyzing the production of the emergent "realities" of these occasions. In order to understand how commitment decisions are accomplished and how hearings are organized, we must first establish the practical purpose and orientations of the hearings from the points of view of their participants. Chapter 3 begins the analysis by considering some of these interpretive orientations.

Notes

1.   It is important to remember that the categorization of persons as mad, insane, mentally ill, and so on was shifting and developing at the same time as treatments evolved. It is extremely difficult to summarize developments in mental health treatment because the concepts of *mental health* and *mental illness* were themselves emerging simultaneously with and reflexively tied to institutionalized responses. We must remember that we are not examining an evolving set of responses to a phenomenon that remained constant while responses developed. To describe the "evolution" of mental health care implies that care was responsive to what was a "medical" problem all along, and that responses to the problem became progressively better informed and more appropriate to their treatment. But, as Foucault (1965) suggests, retrospective analysis from the current perspective of "madness as mental illness" privileges a way of constituting the phenomenon in a way that denies the sociohistorical location and character of the constituting practices. But, of course, Foucault falls victim to the same problem as he attempts to fashion his own history of "insanity" or "madness."

2.   After the initial fourteen-day confinement, persons certified as mentally disordered and gravely disabled may be certified for an additional thirty-day temporary conservatorship for evaluation and review. A judicial hearing is then held to determine if the conservatorship should be made "permanent." Permanent conservatorships are technically for one-year periods that are indefinitely renewable by mandatory annual judicial review. Conservatees are entitled to judicial review every six months. Conservatorship represents the longest term detention of the mentally disordered and places conservatees' property as well as their liberty under the control of their conservators. Conservators may place conservatees in their own homes, nursing homes, board and care facilities, private psychiatric facilities, or public hospitals, so that conservatorship may amount to extended involuntary commitment in some instances.

3.   All names of persons and places have been fictionalized to safeguard the identities of those studied.

4.   In one study site, a court commissioner rather than a judge presided over "possible cause" hearings (after two- or three-day evaluation holds) but a judge conducted hearings involving longer commitments.

5.   As a part of a related project studying community mental health services, colleagues of mine interviewed judges, mental patients, mental health workers, and others who may have experienced aspects of the commitment process. Audiotape recordings of some of these interviews provide information that I have also used to a very limited extent in this study.

6.   Technically, these witnesses were not always psychiatrists; some were psychologists or MDs. For convenience I will hereinafter refer to all such witnesses as *psychiatrists* even though this may not be literally the case. All were certified to give psychiatric testimony.

7.   An occasion when a substitute judge came to Metropolitan Court for several days illustrates the importance of these tacit agreements and routines for

maintaining the efficiency of the court. On his first morning in court, the new judge noted that a psychiatrist called to the witness stand was not the treating psychiatrist in the case being considered. He was somewhat perplexed at the DA's hurried explanation that the PD's office routinely stipulated that other doctors familiar with the case would be allowed to testify. Citing his unfamiliarity with commitment procedures, the judge said he was going to have to go "by the book" and observe the law as he understood it. In the absence of the treating physician, he said, he was granting the writ—that is, terminating the hearing, and thus the commitment.

For the remainder of the morning session, the PDs challenged the testimony of each psychiatrist, and writs were granted each time the treating psychiatrist was not present. In those hearings that did go forward, PDs began to object to "hearsay" testimony, even though the DAs attempted to explain to the judge that hearsay was typically admissible if it were cited as the basis for making a psychiatric evaluation. The judge was unimpressed, and refused to allow the testimony.

By the end of the morning, all writs had been granted—perhaps a dozen in all. There was no need for an afternoon session. The attorneys from the PD's office were having difficulty disguising their amusement over the sudden wealth of "winning" cases, while the DAs fumed over what they perceived as the judge's incompetence and the betrayal by their PD counterparts. The judge was bewildered. After the courtroom emptied, he remained seated at the bench, head in hands. I was the only person remaining in the courtroom, furtively working on my field notes, paying little attention to the judge. Although he had never seen me before, the judge looked out at me and helplessly asked, "What in the hell is going on here?" not really expecting an answer, but looking for some clue as to why the court had fallen into such disarray.

By the next morning, after several phone calls and meetings, the court returned to a semblance of its normal routine—although much more formal, and with many more interruptions by the judge, questioning the legal bases for what was transpiring before him. While he granted a higher than normal percentage of writs, the judge managed to survive his temporary assignment, and hearings became, once again, relatively routine.

8.   Official transcriptions of court proceedings were always recorded in all the courts I studied. In some instances I had access to some of these, but they were not routinely typed up and duplicated, much less circulated. More importantly, officially produced transcriptions are heavily edited throughout the recording process. Statements made, but known to be "off the record," would not appear in official transcripts, for example. Nor would the exact wording of many segments of talk. For my analytic purposes, my own near-transcriptions were superior to officially produced documents.

Chapter 3

Decision-Making in Context: Outlook and Orientations

Involuntary commitment proceedings provoke collisions between medical, legal, and humanitarian concerns. Consider the diverse issues raised in the following exchange between a DA and a psychiatrist who has been called to testify that patient Howard Kimel should be committed.

[3:1]   [Metropolitan Court; J1, DA2, PD5, Dr8, Howard Kimel][1]

DA2:   Are you familiar with the provisions of Lanterman-Petris-Short?

Dr8:   Yes I am.

DA2:   And are you familiar with the patient, Howard Kimel?

Dr8:   Yes, I interviewed him at intake and have examined him several times after his admission.

DA2:   As a result of these examinations have you formulated a diagnosis?

Dr8:   Schizophrenia, chronic undifferentiated.

DA2:   So you believe that the patient suffers from a mental disorder?

Dr8:   Yes, he has a long history of mental illness . . .

DA2:   Now, in your opinion, would you say that Mr. Kimel is gravely disabled as a result of this mental disorder?

Dr8:   Yes, I'd have to say so. He's unable to provide adequate nutrition. He doesn't take care of himself, has nowhere to stay. He does bizarre things, disruptive things for no apparent reason. . . . He wanders from place to place, no home, no family, no permanent address. . . . He has no income, no job. He's mentally ill, and he can't provide for himself in his present condition. It's a clear case of gravely disabled. If he doesn't receive further treatment, he will certainly deteriorate, get even worse.

DA2:   So, you believe that Mr. Kimel meets the standards of LPS and should remain in the hospital.

Dr8:   That's my opinion.

Here, as in nearly all aspects of commitment proceedings, the discourses of mental health and illness, psychiatric treatment, and judicial oversight merge to produce descriptions and decisions that are both medically informed and legally accountable. But the proceedings also orient to commonsense assumptions about everyday life that most people hold, assumptions that make them members of a community of meaning. Because they involve public interpretations of what is normal and abnormal, typical and atypical, competent and incompetent, commitment proceedings provide a rich opportunity to witness and explicate the interpretive practices that produce the everyday world as we know it.

Contingent Factors and Commitment Decisions

While involuntary commitment laws ostensibly govern the commitment process, those laws must be concretely implemented; the law must be articulated with the practical features of the case at hand. For example, in California, LPS clearly states that a person must, as a result of mental disorder, be a danger to others, or him- or herself, or gravely disabled in order to be involuntarily detained and treated. While this may sound straightforward, its application is not clear-cut. The law cannot specify how it might be applied in each instance of its possible use. Nor can it designate those occasions when its use is appropriate. Its application is a practical, interpretive matter.

The questions this chapter attempts to answer concern the contextual factors and contingencies that influence commitment proceedings and decisions. Rather than ask if the law is properly observed or implemented, the analysis asks, To what do commitment hearing participants orient as they conduct their public deliberations? The concern is not so much with the proper application of the law as with the ways in which the law is *used* in the practical context of commitment decision-making. The analysis takes the position that persons invoke and elaborate laws, rules, normative standards, and the like in conjunction with specific cases in order to show how their own actions and decisions are rational, coherent, precedented, and so forth (Zimmerman and Wieder 1970). The law is thus analyzed as a resource for making decisions "accountable." As Warren (1982) suggests, commitment hearings are public occasions where justice is "seen to be done."

But the law is merely one contingent factor in the commitment process. The academic controversy over involuntary commitment decisions points to the possibility that extralegal and nonpsychiatric factors may also influence the commitment process (see Hiday 1988 for a comhensive review of empirical research on civil commitment). A number of studies suggest that specific psychiatric conditions seem to be associated with decisions to commit (Gove 1980; Hiday 1983). Others note that dangerous, assaultive, delusional, or hallucinating candidate patients are most likely to be committed (Hiday 1983; Stoffelmayr, Roth, Parker, and Dillavou 1988; Warren 1982). Personal characteristics like candidate patients' race (Nicholson 1986; Rosenfield 1984; Warren 1982), gender (Horwitz 1982; Nicholson 1986; Rosenfield 1984), age (Haney and Michielutte 1968; Haney et al. 1969; Nicholson 1986), education (Nicholson 1986), and physical appearance (Warren 1982) have been linked to hearing outcomes. Candidate patients' financial and social network resources (Nicholson 1986; Thompson and Ager 1988) and socioeconomic status (Linsky 1970a, 1970b; Rushing 1971) have also been associated with commitment decisions. And finally, some studies suggest that candidate patients with prior psychiatric hospitalizations, those who refuse to take medications or who have been unreliable in outpatient treatment, and candidate patients who have been unable to take care of themselves outside the hospital are likely to be committed (Bursztajn, Gutheil, Mills, Hamm, and Brodsky 1986; Stoffelmayr et al. 1988; Warren 1982).

A range of factors not directly related to candidate patient characteristics has also been associated with commitment decisions. These include the path of entry into commitment proceedings (Belcher 1988; Durham, Carr, and Pierce 1984; Rosenfield 1984), the type of person initiating commitment proceedings (Haney and Michielutte 1968), the diligence of the petitioner in pursuing commitment (Wilde 1968), the presence of an attorney representing the candidate patient at commitment hearings (Wenger and Fletcher 1969), the willingness of family members to accept and care for candidate patients in the home (Greenley 1972; Hiday 1983; Steadman and Cocozza 1974; Warren 1982), and the rate of locally available psychiatric inpatient care openings (Belcher 1988; Haney and Michielutte 1968).

Unfortunately, many findings have been equivocal. Others have been contradicted. Haney and Michielutte (1968), for example, argue that candidate patients' age is strongly related to judgments of mental incompetence, a prerequisite for involuntary commitment. Other studies, however, find no relation between age and commitment decisions (Appelbaum and Hamm 1982; Hiday 1983). Indeed, Hiday (1983) finds no relation between commitment decisions and candidate patients' race, sex, or age. Other findings are equally contradictory and puzzling.

Generally, the studies reviewed here conceive of the potentially influential factors as fixed variables that are contingent aspects of commitment cases. Studies of gender effects on commitment decisions, for example, have typically assumed that a candidate patient's sex is an intrinsic and immutable feature of the person that potentially influenced commitment decisions. Conceiving of commitment procedures in terms of interpretive practice, however, suggests that gender, like other characteristics, is an emergent feature of its social context (Gerson and Peiss 1985). Contingent factors like age, gender, and race become influential through the ways in which they are invoked, made salient, and oriented to. Consequently, the relevance of any particular factor might not be found in its mere presence, but rather in the ways that it is *made* relevant in the discourse of commitment proceedings.

So, rather than inspect commitment proceedings for the relative presence or absence of these and other factors, and attempt to measure their influence on commitment decisions, this analysis focuses on how factors are *made* salient, important, and consequential through the interactional proceedings themselves. In this fashion, we can examine if and how the myriad factors suggested by prior research, and others yet to be noticed, may be introduced into the commitment process.

Background Assumptions and Orientations

While commitment proceedings provide a measure of due process and advocacy (Decker 1987), they hardly resemble criminal or civil proceedings where legal adversaries single-mindedly contest case outcomes (Warren 1982). Several interpretive concerns shape the proceedings, moderating adversarial relations, relaxing judicial and legal procedures, and influencing the ways that participants formulate commitment arguments and decisions.

Mental Illness Assumptions

Nearly everyone involved with the involuntary commitment proceedings I observed believes that persons whose commitment is under consideration are mentally ill—a working assumption that other studies of contemporary commitment proceedings have also noted (Hiday 1983; Warren 1982). Courtroom personnel—including judges and patients' attorneys—anticipate that persons brought before the court will be severely disturbed. In part, this reflects their experience that anyone advancing to a commitment hearing has already been thoroughly screened by the mental health system. Moreover, because commitment cannot even be considered without evidence of profound mental disturbance, the psychiatric testimony at commitment hearings invariably certifies persons sought to be committed as mentally ill. These diagnoses are very rarely challenged by defense attorneys or patients.

According to courtroom personnel, direct experience with patients confirms the psychiatric testimony. One Metropolitan Court judge, for example, indicated that "I know all of these people—every one of them—have problems. That's why they're here. Most are very, very sick." A judge from another jurisdiction somewhat less tactfully suggested that "Everyone of them that comes through here is crazy in one way or another." Informally, nearly all courtroom personnel use terms like *crazy, loony, nuts, unbalanced,* or *ready for the nuthouse* to characterize proposed patients. This is even true (perhaps especially true) of representatives of the PD's office, who are ostensibly arguing for the release of the very people they refer to as *weirdos, nut cases, insane,* and the like.

Nearly everyone also assumes that patients' psychological afflictions are chronic; they view their lives as ongoing "careers" in mental illness. The general feeling is that there is little hope for cure or recovery. Symptoms episodically arise and abate in a cycle of acute disturbance, remission, then relapse. While such prognoses are not optimistic, the personnel involved in commitment proceedings generally believe that psychiatric treatment and therapies are beneficial, if only in containing symptoms of psychological distress. They are aware, however, of the shortcomings and side effects of most conventional treatments, so one seldom hears anyone connected with commitment proceedings arguing that commitment or psychiatric treatment of any sort might effectively cure psychiatric problems, or even contain them for an extended period. In short, court personnel and others involved in commitment proceedings tend to assess patients and the psychiatric services being offered to them in ways reminiscent of members of the psychiatric community themselves. Their commonsense model of craziness or insanity resembles the medical model of psychiatric disturbance, but is articulated in more familiar, less technical vernacular terms. Commitment proceedings, then, are very much concerned with the issues of insanity or craziness, as practical descriptive categories that must mesh with the legal categories to which proceedings orient.[2]

Despite the skeptical (some would say realistic) view of patients' conditions and chances for recovery, some type of psychiatric intervention is nearly always preferred to inaction or benign neglect. In particular, court personnel generally feel that psychotropic medications can be used to stabilize the behavior of persons in the midst of acute episodes and to prolong periods of remission. Finally, while judges and others involved in commitment proceedings believe that mental illness causes persons to behave strangely or irrationally, they nonetheless acknowledge that patients—no matter how "sick"—are periodically capable of lucid, reasonable behavior. "You can get them up there on the stand and they are just as reasonable as you and me," noted one judge. "It doesn't last, but they can pull it together from time to time." In addition, most feel that mental illness does not completely incapacitate its victims, even the chronically afflicted; it may affect only certain behavioral or cognitive realms, impairing some faculties only slightly or sporadically. Nevertheless, when patients comport themselves in a reasonable, competent manner, others involved in commitment proceedings are likely to regard this "normalcy" as a charade—a hoax perpetrated by a crazy person in order to secure one more chance at freedom.

While past research has been concerned with establishing candidate patients' psychiatric condition independently from the assessments used in actual commitment proceedings, my analysis focuses on members' practical, working definitions. I treat mental illness as something that participants in commitment hearings believe is real; they construe its presence as an objective feature of the persons whose commitment is under consideration. My analysis will try to explicate the ways that the "practical reality" of mental illness—as it is known and acted upon by participants—influences the commitment process.

Organizational Orientations

A variety of persons are involved in producing commitment decisions, though some of them seldom appear in court. The persons whose commitment is under consideration generally come to commitment hearings via the mental health care system, frequently with long histories of both out- and inpatient care in a variety of psychiatric settings. Physicians, psychiatrists, psychologists, social workers, and other psychiatric and social service personnel and agencies have invariably been involved in screening, treating, and caring for patients as part of the statutorily mandated procedures for involuntary detention and treatment. Patients are also likely to have encountered law enforcement personnel, often during episodes that precipitate commitment proceedings. These actors constitute an interorganizational network within which commitment decisions are made and to which commitment hearings orient (Warren 1982).

In most jurisdictions, the legal, psychiatric, and social service personnel routinely work with each other, developing working relationships that transcend any particular case. While this clearly contributes to the shared assumptions, definitions, and descriptions of mental illness, it also creates a common orientation to the task at hand. As Blumberg (1967) suggests of criminal courts, commitment proceedings transpire in a rather "closed community," where the patient is something of an outsider, both in terms of organizational station and by virtue of his or her presumed mental illness. This has two important and related consequences. First, a sense of local professional or bureaucratic community develops, built on cooperation between members. The result is a routine mode of processing cases that keeps the business of the courts and related agencies flowing relatively smoothly. Warren (1982) suggests that a mood of "we all work together here" sets the tone for dealings in Metropolitan Court; similar cooperative outlooks prevail in other commitment settings as well.

Second, commitment hearing personnel are aware of the interorganizational matrix within which commitment proceedings take place. They share a set of presumptions about what has already been done to and for the patient, as well as what options remain open. They recognize policies and practices of the various actors in the mental health care and legal systems, and anticipate the repercussions of commitment decisions for both patients and the agencies patients might encounter, depending upon the court's decision. This results in a shared sense of the available possibilities for any particular case.

Like other social control agents, court personnel employ a justificatory decision logic regarding coercive responses to the mentally ill that frames civil commitment as a remedy of "last resort" (Emerson 1981, 1989; Warren 1982). Judges appear keenly aware of this, assuming that the court is, in a sense, insulated by several layers of organizational procedures to which apparently disturbed persons are subjected before involuntary commitment is sought. These persons' troubles come to be understood by reference to remedial efforts that are presumed to have been tried. Commitment is seen as a viable option only if the patient is severely ill, this illness has been repeatedly confirmed elsewhere, and a number of other less coercive and restrictive interventions have been tried and have failed. Consequently, court personnel, like others in the mental health care system, typically look for less intrusive options that might be tried before commitment must be sought.

These concerns combine in a way that often leaves participants in commitment hearings in something short of adversarial positions regarding hearing outcomes. Most participants rely upon the smooth operation of the system to permit them to do their jobs efficiently and effectively. Adversary confrontation over issues about which they generally agree would serve only to complicate their work. And, despite a seeming insensitivity to the psychological distress plaguing most patients, most court personnel do care about what happens to the patients. Indeed, on some occasions they appear more concerned with securing patients' well-being and "best interests" than they are with providing uncompromised legal advocacy or aggressive "prosecution." In a sense, this is a further manifestation of "working together" in commitment proceedings to accomplish a common goal.

Promoting Patients' "Best Interests"

The mental illness assumption provides an interpretive background against which an "interventionist" orientation to mental health problems was maintained in the courts studied. Courtroom personnel generally preferred resolutions that attempted to do something for the patient, to contain or remedy the problems at hand. Any decision rendered—even decisions to release—were apt to be characterized as measures taken on the patient's behalf. Judges invariably argued that "sick" or "crazy" people needed help, noting that "we have to do whatever is best for these troubled people," and "we have to do something, anything, to help the poor souls, or they'll just get worse." The result was a persistent orientation to a case's distinctive "remedial horizons" (Emerson 1981).

Generally, hospitalization was framed as a remedy that, in the words of a Metropolitan Court judge, provides the opportunity "to get people back on the right track, straighten them out, get them stabilized, and get them under control. Then they can go out and stay out for a little bit longer." Hospital stays were depicted as integral parts of mental illness careers, and although repeated admissions stood as evidence of hospitalization's ineffectiveness in curing mental illness, the notion persisted that severe disturbances would proliferate and endure without it. One Northern Court judge summarized this position: "They never get well, but if they don't get help—someone always looking after them, medication, therapy, trips to the hospital—they will always fall back."

Arranging the most desirable outcome for everyone concerned often involves negotiations vaguely resembling the plea bargaining that takes place in criminal courts. In all of the jurisdictions studied, even the PDs, who ostensibly represented patients' interest in avoiding commitment were just as anxious to see some of their clients hospitalized, as were the DAs and psychiatrists who opposed them in court. To this end, PDs often employed a variety of informal practices to arrange treatment and custody while circumventing actual commitment decisions. While several studies (Gilboy and Schmidt 1971; Lewis, Goetz, Schoenfield, Gordon, and Griffin 1984; Miller, Maher, and Fiddleman 1984) imply that candidate patients are often coerced into such arrangements, I never encountered evidence that patients were forced to forfeit their rights to court hearings. Nonetheless, it was clear in all the jurisdictions I studied that avoiding involuntary commitments was a high priority for nearly everyone involved.

For example, staff members at psychiatric facilities often tried vigorously to persuade patients who were confined on emergency admissions to sign "voluntary" admission papers in order to facilitate "necessary" treatment, but also to avoid the administrative difficulties associated with habeas corpus proceedings. Their persuasive tactics might include implying that criminal charges could be filed and imprisonment might result from disturbances associated with the emergency hospitalizations. In other instances, patients might be told that they could "check out" anytime they wanted if they agreed to a voluntary admission, but that an involuntary commitment could result in long-term confinement. In one jurisdiction, staff in the state psychiatric facility housing many involuntary patients suggested that patients would receive better treatment, with extended freedom and privileges, if they were voluntarily admitted.

As cases moved toward formal commitment proceedings, court personnel often took up the challenge of reaching a "reasonable disposition" of a case that would keep a patient under supervision and treatment without resorting to formal involuntary commitment. Even PDs often believed that arguing strongly on behalf of a client's desire for release was not always in the client's best interest. Often their contact with delusional or nonresponsive clients convinced PDs that further hospitalization and treatment was clearly in order. In most such instances, they tried to convince their clients that further hospitalization and treatment was the best course to pursue, and occasionally they went to great lengths to prevent their clients from going forward with formal hearings.

For instance, one PD in Metropolitan Court capitalized on her client's "delusional" state of mind to extract an agreement to stay in the hospital and voluntarily drop his request for a hearing. The client, Patrick Claire, a white male perhaps forty years old, was seated in the hallway outside the courtroom when he beckoned Joan Kingman, a PD who was apparently trying to find a client she was supposed to represent later that day. Mr. Claire very politely and directly asked Ms. Kingman if she was a lawyer, or "one of those shrinks." Kingman asked Mr. Claire who he was, and was only slightly taken aback when he replied "You mean you don't recognize the president of the United States?" Kingman apologized and excused herself momentarily. After glancing at one of the files she was carrying, she turned back and asked, "You wouldn't be Patrick Claire, would you?" "They keep saying so, but I'll not hear of it," replied Mr. Claire. The PD then returned to the man's original question, telling

Mr. Claire that she was a lawyer, in fact, the attorney appointed to represent him in his commitment hearing that afternoon. Mr. Claire, clearly pleased, drew her close and, in a conspiratorial tone, offered her a proposition.

[3:2]   [Metropolitan Court; PD5, Patrick Claire]

> You know that as president, I can do your career quite a favor. You get me out of this [hospitalization], and I'll fix you up. Jack Kennedy gets his way around Washington, you know. You work something out, and I'll name you attorney general. Bobby [Kennedy] wants to run for senator, so I'll need someone to take over. You show me you're a good lawyer and you've got the job.

The conversation continued for several minutes, with the client repeatedly asserting that he was President Kennedy, even as the PD reminded him that Kennedy had died twenty years before. Several times Ms. Kingman suggested to Mr. Claire that perhaps "it would be best in the long run if you took a little more time off" in the hospital. She finally excused herself, sought out a representative of the DA's office, and told him that she had a "difficult" case on her hands. She inquired about the argument the DA was going to make, and was told that the testifying psychiatrist was adamant that Mr. Claire was actively schizophrenic, with severe delusions and other florid symptoms. The DA was going to argue that Mr. Claire was gravely disabled, and he felt confident that the judge would deny the writ and continue the hospitalization "unless you [the PD] throw a wrench in the gears."

The PD assured the DA that she had no intention of doing anything but letting "President Kennedy" testify on his own behalf. She then returned to Mr. Claire and asked him once more if he wouldn't reconsider dropping his petition for a court hearing. Finally, with somewhat exaggerated concern in her voice, Kingman pleaded:

[3:3]   [Metropolitan Court; PD5, Patrick Claire]

> Mr. President, if you go through with this hearing, it will end your political career. Just think what people would think—the president in court to see if he needs to be locked in a mental asylum. Even if I get you out, you're finished politically. Think about it. But if you take a few more days in the hospital, a week or two maybe, you can say it's just for a rest, you know, recuperation from the stresses of the presidency. No one needs to find out.

Mr. Claire paused for a moment, then conceded: "OK, let's do it, but let's keep this whole thing quiet." The PD hurried off to find the psychiatrist from the facility treating Mr. Claire to ask him to get Claire back to the ward as quickly as possible, while she informed the court that the writ had been dropped.

While not a typical case, nor a typical way of representing a client, this illustrates the commonly spoken preference of court personnel—PDs included—for working out "reasonable" dispositions rather than insisting on adversarial hearings and judicial decisions. Indeed, several PDs and three of the judges studied explicitly noted that they thought that they should make every effort to avoid commitment proceedings. As one PD suggested, "I'm here to provide legal counsel and representation, but I also think I should be doing all I can to prevent these hearings." A judge expressed a similar view:

[3:4] [Metropolitan Court; J2]

> Patients have many rights, and they shouldn't lose their freedom arbitrarily, but sometimes it's probably not a good thing for them to exercise all those rights. They're better off if they get some treatment, even if they might not be technically committable.

The prevailing sentiment articulated by court personnel, then, combined a concern with judicial oversight with a desire to see troubled persons get the care they were thought to need. PDs, DAs, and judges frequently cooperated to get patients into treatment, actively negotiating resolutions that they believed were best for the patients involved. Of course, this often meant that patients' opinions and desires were viewed skeptically, if not disregarded. Another instance from Metropolitan Court is illustrative.

When PD Lena Gray interviewed her client in the hall outside the courtroom, she found Jerome Snow, a white male in his twenties, to be almost incommunicative. He was attentive and compliant, but answered only a few of her questions, generally with single-word answers. Mr. Snow's mother was with him that day, and after Ms. Gray concluded her talk with Mr. Snow, Mrs. Snow took Ms. Gray aside and pleaded with her to find a way to keep her son in the hospital for a little while longer. Ms. Gray told Mrs. Snow that she was Mr. Snow's attorney and it was her job to make sure his wishes were represented, that she could not act against his wishes.

As Ms. Gray excused herself, DA Tom Adler approached and told Ms. Gray, "This guy [Mr. Snow] is going back [is going to be committed]. His mother wants to make a fuss, and he's clearly a pretty disturbed guy." Ms. Gray agreed, but said that Mr. Snow wanted to go ahead with the hearing: "He says he doesn't want to spend any more time in the hospital." "I'll tell ya," replied Mr. Adler, "he's better off without the hearing, because Mom says she'll be up to handling him in a few days, but if we commit him, he's gone for longer than that."

Mr. Adler then offered a suggestion. Rather than risk an additional fourteen-day confinement, he asked Ms. Gray if she couldn't talk Mr. Snow into admitting himself voluntarily until his mother agreed to let him come home. He said this would save everyone a lot of trouble. Mr. Adler indicated that the judge was concerned that Mr. Snow might be committed today, but his mother might soon change her mind and agree that he could come home. Mr. Snow would then be back in court again, in two weeks if not a couple of days. Ms. Gray thought Mr. Adler's suggestion sounded reasonable, so she said she would talk to the Snows once more.

Returning to where the Snows were now seated, Ms. Gray approached Mr. Snow. "You know, Jerome, your parents are worried about you. They think you should stay in the hospital for a little while longer." Mr. Snow smiled weakly, but shook his head no. "You can go in and ask the judge if you can go home if you want," Ms. Gray continued, "and I'll help you if you want, but I think you should think about it. Your parents are worried about you. Think about it. What if you had a child who had problems?" Mr. Snow continued to shake his head. Ms. Gray persisted: "If you stay in the hospital, they can help you. A little while longer and they'll have you stabilized and then it will be all right for you to come home. That's what your parents want. For you to get the treatment you really need." Mr. Snow just smiled.

Ms. Gray made one final attempt at persuasion: "If you admit yourself to the hospital on your own, you can sign yourself out any time you want, Jerome. But if you don't, you might have to stay for at least another two weeks." Mr. Snow asked Ms. Gray to repeat this, and she went on to explain voluntary admission procedures. She then suggested that Mr. Snow was almost surely going to be committed, and then he would be in the hospital longer than if he admitted himself with an agreement to go home once his mother was ready for him and his medication had stabilized his condition. Finally, without emotion, Mr. Snow told Ms. Gray that he didn't want to see the judge, that he would drop the writ and go back to the hospital. Ms. Gray told him he was doing the right thing, then went into the courtroom to find Mr. Snow's doctor to arrange his voluntary admission.

Instances like this display both the general concern for patients' best interest (regardless of what the patient might say), and court personnel's desire to work together to accomplish the court's goals and conduct business as efficiently as possible. While this means that patients' expressed wishes were often ignored or manipulated, many hearings and involuntary commitments were avoided.

The desire to see that patients received needed treatment was evident in several related ways. In one jurisdiction, PDs who felt their clients needed extended treatment would ask that their cases be "continued in order to properly prepare." This was a legitimate legal maneuver, and routinely produced delays of up to ten days that could be used to provide treatment that might stabilize patients. Indeed, this length of time closely corresponded to the time local psychiatrists believed was necessary to "saturate" patients with psychoactive medications, then begin to reduce dosages in order to find a manageable maintenance dosage.

In what they perceived as extreme cases, PDs—often in a sort of collusion with the judge and DA—could all but ensure a decision to commit by allowing a client to present his or her case for release in such a way as to display mental disturbance and interactional inappropriateness, tacitly corroborating the testimony from their clients that would prove damaging to their pleas for release. For example, clients might be asked questions that provided the occasion for displays of "delusions" or other "unreasonable" claims, stories, and descriptions. Or PDs might underscore the implausibility of their clients' claims by ironically summarizing problematic statements as if they were unimpeachable arguments for release. The following illustration shows a PD, in ironic, almost sarcastic tones, reiterating his client's claims for the judge. The patient had testified that he had no mental problems and could provide for all his basic needs because he had a "benefactor" who let him stay in his hotel room. The client said he had all the food and clothing he needed right there in the courtroom with him, indicating a large plastic garbage bag full of clothing and other odds and ends. The PD summarized his client's testimony:

[3:5] [Metropolitan Court; J1, DA2, PD3, Dr11, Russel Howard]

> You can see, your honor, that my client is doing perfectly well. There is no basis whatsoever for certifying him as gravely disabled. He's obviously fine. He's got his complete fall wardrobe right there with him in that plastic bag. His lunch is in his pocket. And we have little reason to believe that he is not welcome to stay at the Airport Hilton anytime he wants . . .

While instances like these are common, they do not mean that PDs abandon their role as their clients' advocates; patients' legal rights and representation were not consistently or completely compromised. To the contrary, on most occasions PDs listened patiently to their clients' stories, discerned their desires, familiarized themselves with the psychiatric and social details of the case, and presented arguments for release professionally and convincingly. Given the size of their caseloads, the extremely limited time they had to meet with clients and concerned others, and the sorts of problems that typically arise when dealing with clients facing commitment hearings, PDs capably managed the ex-

tremely tenuous and difficult position by trying to use their legal expertise and position to serve their clients in ways they believed were both
humane and respectful of clients' legal rights. Literally thousands of
cases were formally processed through the court during the years of this
study, and about half of all commitment hearings across all jurisdictions
studied resulted in release. But aggressive advocacy and adversarial zeal
were sometimes subordinated to what court personnel argued were
more important and humane goals.

Psychiatry and the Law

An underlying tension between psychiatry and the law pervades involuntary commitment proceedings. Judges routinely displayed their
concern that decisions were both legally and medically warranted. On
one hand, they deferred to psychiatric personnel regarding diagnostic
matters, generally conceding that such issues were beyond their expertise. They often suggested, however, that psychiatrists were insensitive
to the human costs of hospitalization, especially in terms of lost liberty
and violated rights. "They want to control people so they can treat them,
and they never see this as anything but good. They don't think about a
person's rights," noted a Metropolitan Court judge.

Balancing legal concerns against medical prerogatives, judges openly,
sometimes militantly, displayed their legal authority by publicly insisting that individual rights be protected and laws be upheld. "These people have rights," a Northern Court judge noted, referring to candidate
patients, "and they must have the benefit of the court's protection, even
if their condition is questionable. I may not always make the best medical decision, but they have rights, and the law must be obeyed." Psychiatric expertise was honored, but judges refused to merely confirm or
passively accept medical opinions, as a Metropolitan Court judge noted:

[3:6]   [Metropolitan Court; J1]

Psychiatrists have their skills, but they also have their own interests in
what happens to patients. Some of them think they are the gifted ones, the
only ones who know anything, the only ones that can help. Now, I can't be
led into their trap. I can't believe everything a doctor says, hook, line and
sinker, just because he's an M.D. He may think he knows it all, but I know
the law, and it's up to me to make sure everything that is done is legal.

While judges generally considered involuntary hospitalization to be a
viable option, they were also reluctant to deprive persons of their liberty
without substantial warrant. Still, judges rarely felt that a patient could

be released back into the situation that initially precipitated commitment proceedings unless some remedial action was taken to change it. Hospitalization, then, was typically warranted as a "last resort," when it could be demonstrated that all other reasonable, less restrictive options had been exhausted (Emerson 1981).

By regularly asserting that commitment decisions were fundamentally legal matters—informed but not determined by psychiatric input—judges both reserved for themselves the ultimate authority as decision-maker and staked claim to their own distinctive and legitimate professional competence. And it was through their ability to invoke non-psychiatric criteria—especially aspects of the law—to differentiate between persons to be hospitalized and those to be released that judges displayed their distinctive, judicial decision-making expertise.

Danger or Disability?

Involuntary commitment can be ordered either on the basis of danger to self or others, or because a person is gravely disabled—or a local variant of that category. Over the course of this study, approximately 90 percent of the patients who had habeas corpus writ hearings in Metropolitan Court had been certified as gravely disabled by the doctor requesting hospitalization. In the cases I observed in other jurisdictions, a similar proportion of cases were heard as matters of danger to self, revolving around the issues implied in the grave disability label—that is, the ability of the person to provide for his or her basic necessities. These findings are similar to the trends Warren (1977, 1982) noted in her earlier studies, where she found grave disability charged in approximately three out of four commitment cases. Commitment on the basis of either dangerousness charge was pursued only in cases where danger to self or others seemed clearly and convincingly documented.

While this preponderance of grave disability charges might be a function of the sorts of psychological and social disturbances exhibited by persons whose commitment was sought, it is also related to the practical circumstances of arguing commitment cases. While judges and DAs note that they regularly pursue the charge that seems most appropriate, they also admit that it is generally easier to "prove" grave disability. To hospitalize a person because he or she has endangered him- or herself typically requires evidence of a recent overt act that was intended to be harmful. Providing such evidence is often difficult, or at least more difficult than arguing that a person is not meeting his or her basic needs. Consequently, DAs encouraged the use of the grave disability criterion whenever feasible.

[3:7] [Metropolitan Court; DA3]

> We always ask the psychiatrist to check grave disability [on hospitalization
> forms]. It's just easier that way. They can ask for certification for danger,
> too, but we need disability. They [psychiatrists] shouldn't care on what
> grounds. They get them in the hospital one way or another. If they don't
> certify gravely disabled, our chances for committing are not too good.
> You've got to have an observed attempt at suicide or mayhem—you know,
> the smoking pistol—or they're going to go free. But if we're arguing dis-
> ability, almost anything goes—anything they do that isn't for their own
> good.

While the standards for proving dangerousness may appear daunting, a wide range of factors was routinely cited as evidence of grave
disability. Giving away money, spending time on the roof, running up a
two-hundred-dollar-a-month water bill by bathing repeatedly, refusing
to eat, failing to cooperate with psychiatric hospital staff and treatment
regimens, and halfheartedly attempting suicide were all argued as examples of inability to adequately care for one's self. "If he can't seem to
make a go of it on the outside, I'll say that he's gravely disabled,"
remarked one judge. "The law has to be flexible." In practice, grave
disability appears to have meaning almost independent of the formal
statute in that it incorporates a wide range of considerations regarding
the patient's welfare in the context of community life. These may include, but not be confined to, the provision of food, clothing, and shelter. If a person is "unable to provide for the basic necessities of life," or is
"unable to take care of himself," according to two judges, he or she is
gravely disabled.

Court personnel may also interpret evidence that seemingly demonstrates danger to self or danger to others as an indication of grave disability. As a DA noted, "We can even make instances of danger into
evidence for disability. Harming one's self isn't taking very good care of
yourself, right?" Even apparent episodes of dangerousness to others can
be argued as proof of disability. For example, one patient in Metropolitan Court was judged gravely disabled in part because he had antag-
onized and assaulted strangers in public places as well as other patients
on his hospital ward. The man was not physically imposing, and in-
flicted no real harm. His psychiatrist and the DA argued that the man
was gravely disabled because his behavior incited others, and their re-
taliations might endanger his welfare.

While DAs may prefer to charge candidate patients with grave disability rather than dangerousness, PDs also prefer this charge from time
to time. A PD in Metropolitan Court, for example, may negotiate an

agreement with a DA and the testifying psychiatrist to have a client certified as gravely disabled rather than as dangerous to others because commitment on the basis of dangerousness can result in a ninety-day detention, rather than the fourteen-day hospitalization for grave disability. Warren (1977, 1982) has characterized such agreements as a "bargaining down" the charges against a person whose commitment is sought. All participants in the hearing receive some ostensible benefit. The PD reduces the chance that the patient will be hospitalized for an extended period; the patient, while committed, will be eligible for release in a matter of days and will not have been labeled as dangerous; the DA ensures that the patient will be hospitalized for treatment; and the judge will not have to adjudicate the difficult issue of imminent and predictable danger.

In one sense, the preponderance of grave disability charges represents another aspect of the ways that court personnel work together to facilitate the court's routines. But my observations also suggest that pursuing commitment on the basis of grave disability—arguing that patients are severely disturbed and consequently not obtaining life's basic necessities—is most often a practical choice made somewhat unilaterally by DAs and consulting psychiatrists who seek the surest way of detaining and treating needy patients. The greater ease in obtaining decisions to commit comes at almost no significant cost. The short commitments granted on the grounds of grave disability provide enough time to begin and stabilize drug treatments, thus satisfying the most pressing interests of the psychiatrists and DAs. While PDs may sometime be enlisted in "bargains" regarding the grounds upon which their clients are being committed, DAs typically seek certification on the grounds of grave disability without consulting the patient or his or her counsel.

A variety of factors, then, affect the commitment process, many of them acting at a distance from the courtroom. Warren (1982) and others have detailed the complex interorganizational matrix that influences who ultimately ends up being committed. Both intra- and interorganizational considerations are consequential to the hearing themselves, if not directly, then in terms of participants' background knowledge and assumptions—frameworks that participants use to interpret the matters they encounter during the hearings.

* * * * *

Background knowledge supplies a set of orientations to commitment issues, but the hearings themselves provide the interactional scaffolding upon which arguments and decisions are built. Chapter 4 begins the analysis of the interactional organization of the hearing process.

Notes

1.   Data extracts will indicate all participants in the hearings from which the conversational data were taken. Each extract will indicate the jurisdiction, the judge (J), district attorney (DA), public defender (PD), psychiatrist (Dr), and patient involved. Examples taken from interviews and other encounters will also indicate jurisdiction and involved participants.

2.   Chapter 7 considers in greater detail the use of the mental illness assumption as an interpretive framework.

Chapter 4

The Sequential Organization of Commitment Hearings

Legal proceedings are designed to produce decisions that are recognizable to participants and observers as more definite, final, binding, and judicious than decisions arrived at by other, informal means (Atkinson and Drew 1979). Legal settings differ from ordinary conversations because special rules and procedures provide ways of dealing with some of the practical problems associated with argumentation and decision-making. For example, courtrooms are multiparty settings involving a variety of speakers, but official procedures indicate the boundaries of the proceedings, specify the parties who may legitimately participate, and predetermine their forms of participation.

Talk in commitment hearings is distinctive because it is procedurally limited to direct and cross-examination of witnesses by PDs, DAs, and judges. While proceedings appear rather informal, speakership rights are nonetheless procedurally allocated. The brief descriptions in previous chapters provide an overview of what goes on in commitment hearings, but it superficially glosses the interactional activities that provide the basis for legally warranted, psychiatrically informed decisions. Close examination of commitment hearings reveals a sequential order to the proceedings—an "interrogatory sequence"—that can be systematically elaborated to achieve the various features that characterize commitment hearings. This sequence—regardless of the specific content of the various arguments that are offered—is the defining characteristic of commitment proceedings. In all the jurisdictions studied, commitment hearings either conformed to this framework, or drew attention to deviations from it.

The following sections describe what is said and what goes on in each component of commitment hearings. The sequence provides the framework within which participants offer testimony and arguments demon-

The Hearing Sequence

(A Discourse Sequence for Commitment Hearings)

I. Summons
II. Psychiatric Assessment
    A. Direct examination of doctor by DA
        1. Display doctor's qualifications
        2. Display doctor's assessment methods
        3. Solicit doctor's psychiatric diagnosis
        4. Solicit doctor's opinion regarding the patient's medico-legal status
    B. Cross-examination of doctor by PD
        1. Further questions regarding the doctor's qualifications
        2. Further questions regarding the doctor's assessment methods
        3. Further questions regarding the doctor's opinion regarding the patient's medicolegal status
    C. Questions from judge
III. Rebuttal
    A. Direct Examination of patient by PD
    B. Cross Examination of patient by DA
    C. Question from judge
IV. Commentary and summation
    A. PD's summary arguments
    B. DA's summary arguments
    C. Judge's questions and clarifications
V. Resolution
    A. Unilateral decision by judge, or
    B. Agreement mediated by judge

strating the hearing's orientation to psychiatric expertise as well as its "legality." Exemplary models of each phase of the sequence are offered in illustration, although few hearings conform in all aspects to the overall model sequence. Complete "near transcriptions" of three hearings appear as appendices at the end of the book: the case involving patients Polly Brown (Appendix 1), Regina Farmer (Appendix 2), and Jason Andro (Appendix 3). Exemplary sections of these cases are frequently cited, and readers are encouraged to examine the complete hearings from which they are drawn.

Delimiting Legal Proceedings: The Summons

Whereas commitment proceedings usually take place in formal court-rooms, the setting alone does not provide the recognizable parameters for the official activity. Alternative activity abounds in the settings where commitment hearings take place, much of it commitment related. But even the nature, topic, or relevance of conversations does not neces-sarily identify what comes to be seen as official commitment proceed-ings. The official business of the court—"for the record"—must be inter-actionally distinguished in order to identify for participants, observers, and official records and other accounts of the proceedings just where the proceedings begin. Metropolitan Court, for example, was the work site for several DAs and PDs, who met with one another, sought out and interviewed clients and psychiatrists, and interacted in other business-related and unrelated matters. Psychiatrists, patients, and observers also "hung out" in and around the courtroom, engaging in multifaceted con-versations bearing on the business matters at hand. While the judge's arrival was the ostensible signal that a court session was about to begin, it alone did not initiate the official proceedings.

Some form of identifiable interactional marker was necessary to es-tablish that formal proceedings had commenced. This was typically achieved when a court clerk (or the judge himself) simply proclaimed that court was in session. The presiding judge might also be announced at this time. Such announcements, while often quite matter-of-fact, served to notify the relevant participants that their business was now to be "officially" discussed and they should make themselves available for the hearing. When the DA, PD, and patient had assembled before the bench, the proceedings would formally begin with the judge indicating that the DA should call his or her witness.

The summons phase of the sequence marks off the official proceed-ings from other court activities as well as from the myriad conversations and activities that may be under way in the courtroom. Although the announcement might not immediately quell other conversations, it serves notice that the focus of the court is now on one particular case and that all other discussions will be offstage, backstage, irrelevant, or inappropriate conversations—at least for the time being. This was espe-cially important for hearings that were not conducted in public court-rooms, where it might be especially difficult to differentiate official dis-cussion of the business at hand from preliminary, exploratory, or off the record discussions. In these cases, the beginning of hearings was often signaled by the judge simply stating, "Let's get this hearing under way," or "Let's get down to business here." Or, without a direct announcement, he might achieve a beginning marker by requesting that someone start the tape recorder that was to record the proceedings, or that the clerk in attendance begin keeping records.

Getting started and showing that business is under way are characteristic features of a variety of multiparty, task-oriented settings (Atkinson and Drew 1979; Dingwall 1980; Vandewater 1983). This work is particularly important in legal circumstances because their activities are intended to be seen as procedurally and legally organized, and they are recognized only when they follow the procedural mandate to maintain a single focus within a strictly observed speakership allocation format. There is a general interactional problem posed for such a format by normal turn-taking conventions in multiparty conversations; any potential participant may compete for speakership at any point when speakership transition is possible. Without modification, the normal, ongoing conversations in the room might fail to coalesce into the interrogatory sequence that is identifiable as a commitment hearing. The goal of generating statutorily relevant arguments and achieving an accountable judicial ruling would be impeded, and the procedural correctness of any decision would not be clearly visible. The orderly management of commitment proceedings could therefore not be achieved without the methodical use of some sort of summons or initiation procedure. Carrying out a commitment hearing in legal fashion thus begins with and relies upon initiation work.

Producing Psychiatric Assessments

The initial testimony phase of commitment hearings begins as the DA calls a psychiatric expert to make a recommendation regarding the release or commitment of the patient. The psychiatrist invariably testified that the patient was mentally ill and met the legal criteria for commitment. Except for rare exceptions, this was the only witness called to make the case for commitment. Producing the visible psychiatric and legal warrant for involuntary commitment typically involved several component activities, each contributing to the psychiatric and legal defensibility of the argument to commit.

Direct Examination: Displaying
Doctors' Qualifications

The DA's direct examination of the psychiatric witness begins with an exchange designed to establish the doctor as an expert who is qualified to advise the court. While these exchanges vary from case to case, the following is fairly typical.[1]

[4:1]   [Metropolitan Court: J1, DA1, PD5, Dr12, Sylvia Winston]

1.	DA1:	Would you please state your name, and spell the last name.
2.	Dr12:	Robert W Williams. W I L L I A M S.
3.	DA1:	Are you a trained physician?
4.	Dr12:	I am. I'm a practicing psychiatrist.
5.	DA1:	And where did you receive your training?
6.	Dr12:	At Western State University School of Medicine.
7.	DA:1:	Where did you do your psychiatric residency, Dr. Williams?
8.	Dr12:	Highland State Hospital.
9.	DA1:	How long have you practiced psychiatry?
10.	Dr12:	Eleven years.
11.	DA1:	Are you licensed?
12.	Dr12:	I am.
13.	DA1:	Certified?
14.	Dr12:	Yes, sir.
15.	DA1:	And where are you currently practicing?
16.	Dr12:	I'm on the staff at Veterans Memorial Hospital.
17.	DA1:	How long have you been there?
18.	Dr12:	Three and a half years this May.
19.	DA1:	Have you ever testified in matters involving involuntary
20.		commitments before, Dr. Williams?
21.	Dr12:	Um hum. Yes I have.
22.	DA1:	Before this court?
23.	Dr12:	No, not here.
24.	DA1:	But you have experience in these matters?
25.	Dr12:	I've done this a number of times in other courts, yes.

The questioning sequence displays the witness's medical background and authority, qualifying him to make the assessments that will subsequently be solicited, and anticipating challenges to the doctor's qualifications. The example above is more elaborate and comprehensive than most done in Metropolitan Court, although such exchanges are not uncommon. Psychiatrists appearing in court for the first time, or those who are not recognized by members of the DA's or PD's staff, are more likely to be questioned at length. In such instances, DAs ask psychiatrists to state their occupations, where they received their professional degrees, details of their employment history, and other related questions.[2] Once these doctors establish themselves as court "regulars," however, their qualifications are typically accepted without further question.

In contrast, psychiatrists who are easily recognized are not questioned at such length, if at all. Several local hospitals assign doctors rotating duty as testifying psychiatrist at Metropolitan Court, so many of the doctors appear several times a month. Doctors involved in involuntary commitments in Eastern Court are also likely to be regular courtroom participants. In these instances, the DA typically asks the PD to "stipulate" to the doctor's qualifications—an explicit agreement that the PD will not raise the doctor's qualifications as an issue in the case at hand. The PD nearly always agrees. Thus, the elaborate display of background and credentials exhibited in extract [4:1] is typically replaced by an exchange like the following.

[4:2]   [Metropolitan Court; J2, DA2, PD2, Dr3, William Clarke]

1.   DA2:   Please state your name.
2.   Dr3:   Anthony Prego.
3.   DA2:   [spoken to PD2] Will you stipulate as to Dr. Prego's
4.   qualifications?
5.   PD2:   Stipulated.

The opening sequence, especially in its elaborate form, accomplishes two features of the psychiatric assessment: (1) it displays the qualifications and credibility of psychiatric witnesses, and (2) it privileges the psychiatric viewpoint. Once ratified as an expert, the psychiatrist serves as an implicit referent to which other witnesses may be compared. Any subsequent disagreement with his or her testimony must implicitly challenge his or her expertise as well as the case-specific psychiatric explanation. In addition, the sequence implicitly underscores and authorizes a psychiatric understanding of the troubles that comprise the case at hand. Establishing the doctor not simply as an expert, but as a *psychiatric* authority, gives special warrant to psychiatric explanations for various "facts" and claims that emerge as the case proceeds. Not only are the doctor's interpretations given special status, but the psychiatric paradigm's way of formulating issues is authorized as the prescribed method for evaluating the persons and behaviors in question. These points will be elaborated in subsequent sections.

Producing a Psychiatric Diagnosis

Next, the witness is asked to offer a psychiatric assessment of the patient. This nearly always involves discussion of the doctor's assessment methods as well as details of his or her diagnosis. Through an almost formulaic series of questions, the DA first asks the psychiatrist about how and how well he or she knows the case in question. This segment of the interrogation amounts to a display of the methods and procedures that the doctor has employed to arrive at a medical opinion on the case at hand. Whereas the sequence varies in minor ways, most instances resemble the following example.

[4:3]   [Metropolitan Court; J1, DA2, PD7, Dr1, Ronald Berker]

1. DA2:   Now, Doctor Hickman, are you familiar with the patient?
2. Dr1:   Yes I am.
3. DA2:   Have you interviewed him?
4. Dr1:   Yes.
5. DA2:   Examined him?
6. Dr1:   Yes I have.
7. DA2:   Have you talked with other people at Metro [the facility
8.   where the patient was hospitalized] about him?
9. Dr1:   Yes.
10. DA2:   Have you reviewed his chart?
11. Dr1:   Yes.
12. DA2:   And have you formed an opinion on the patient's mental status?
13. Dr1:   Yes I have.

The sequence lays out the defensible grounds for claiming that the doctor is professionally familiar with the patient and his case. The questioning reveals a systematic and professionally adequate procedure for generating the psychiatric evaluation that will subsequently be solicited. If this is not done, the PD will subsequently ask a similar series of questions, more skeptically framed, to explore the possibility that the witness is not professionally acquainted with the case at hand.

Next, the DA solicits a diagnosis and asks for further display of the procedures and reasoning that lead to the assessment.

[4:4]   [Metropolitan Court; J1, DA2, PD7, Dr1, Ronald Berker]

1. DA2:   What is your diagnosis, doctor?
2. Dr1:   The patient is a chronic schizophrenic, undifferentiated
3.   type.
4. DA2:   And what fact, what set of facts brought him to the hospital?
5. Dr1:   He was shouting and screaming in the middle of rush-hour
6.   traffic. He was out of his car, trying to stop traffic,
7.   direct traffic. When the police brought him in he
8.   wasn't coherent. Admissions couldn't understand him.
9. DA2:   How has his behavior been in the hospital?

10.	Dr1:	He's been confused and disoriented, guarded, suspicious,
11.		withdrawn. He's made several bizarre claims. He tells us
12.		he's a veteran but he's not according to our records.
13.		He's had hallucinations. ((silence))

Here, the doctor specifies his technical assessment of the patient, describing both the circumstances that brought the patient to the attention of psychiatric personnel and the characteristics and behaviors that were considered as the basis for the diagnosis. At this juncture in nearly every hearing, the doctor recites the "symptoms" that have led to the conclusion that the patient was severely mentally ill. In extract [4:4], a specific incident illustrating florid symptoms (the traffic incident), as well as descriptions of more generalized problems ("He's had hallucinations.") are offered as grounds for the diagnosis of chronic schizophrenia.

The explanation of the diagnosis is clearly rhetorical, typically relying upon two components: generalized accounts of the patient's disturbed mental state, and vivid depictions of specific bizarre incidents and/or instances of unconventional behavior. Descriptions like *delusional, violent, paranoid, dangerously aggressive,* and other vernacular, quasi-professional, or technical designations provide a global picture of the patient, establishing traits that are argued to be characteristic of the person evaluated. The descriptions are typically tied to depictions of arguably bizarre activities, conduct, or claims that are cited as documents of the more general problem: The patient "attacked his mother and father with a knife, claiming they were 'Iranian agents'"; the patient said she was a "famous movie star" and was rich enough to "buy this whole hospital"; the patient "said he saw people planning to attack him on the television camera in his head"; the patient claimed to be Jesus Christ, John F. Kennedy, Janis Joplin, Monty Hall, and so forth. The specific instances provide the warrant for the more general characterizations. While not explicitly argued as such, they are the evidence supporting the diagnostic claims. This intent is to provide an unequivocal, substantiated argument that shows beyond question that there is good reason for the diagnosis.

The diagnostic sequence is a sort of psychiatric denunciation, in that the patient is characterized comprehensively, focusing on his or her problematic traits and behaviors as distinguishing attributes, while ignoring aspects of the patient that might be construed as normal. It is characteristic of denunciations that they aim to portray one's character as totally and fundamentally of a particular discredited type (Emerson 1969). While all description is unavoidably selective, the psychiatric assessments are notable for their singular focus on the most extreme qualities of the persons being evaluated, a rhetorically useful maneuver.

Formulating Medicolegal Assessments

Being mentally ill is merely necessary, but not sufficient grounds for involuntary commitment. Evidence of danger or disability due to mental illness is also mandated, so the interrogation of the psychiatric witness typically attempts to link the medical assessment and diagnosis to the legal rubrics under which involuntary hospitalization can be ordered. The following example is typical of questioning sequences designed to elicit the doctor's *medicolegal* assessment of the patient.

[4:5]   [Metropolitan Court; J1, DA2, PD7, Dr1, Ronald Berker]

```
 1.  DA2:  Now, in your opinion, doctor has [Mr. Berker's]
 2.         mental condition left the patient gravely disabled? That is,
 3.         do you feel he is unable to provide for his food, clothes,
 4.         and shelter?
 5.  Dr1:  Yes he is gravely disabled so he can't function socially.
 6.  DA2:  And what leads you to that conclusion?
 7.  Dr1:  The patient has no social skills and is very disorganized
 8.         in public situations. He has trouble with the most routine
 9.         matters that he has to deal with in his daily life, and in my
10.         opinion will not be able to adequately provide for himself.
11.         (He can't interact with other people lucidly.) I can't imagine
12.         that he could buy, him trying to buy food, or keeping track of
13.         his money. He doesn't even know if he has money, as far as I
14.         can tell from talking to him. (If he's released, he's going to
15.         have trouble making it from day to day.) His illness will
16.         make it impossible for him provide for himself, to survive.
```

Note how the DA embedded a legal definition of grave disability into his inquiry. Whereas his recycling and specification (lines 3–4) of his initial question (lines 1–2) might be seen as an effort to merely simplify and clarify, it also outlines the legal criteria for hospitalization in the context of asking whether the criteria had been met. The assessment is elicited, while at the same time the doctor's proper understanding of the meaning of grave disability is made apparent.

As with the psychiatric diagnosis, the DA also asks the doctor to display the grounds for hospitalizing the patient. This portion of the sequence often reiterates the factors assimilated to the psychiatric diagnosis, using similar rhetorical technique but stressing the ways in which the "symptoms" of the diagnosed mental illness render the patient either dangerous to him- or herself or others, or precludes the person from providing for his or her food, clothing, shelter, or other daily necessities. In extract [4:5], for instance, the doctor describes some of the patient's troubles (lines 7–8), and then indicates how they will pose difficulties along lines specified by LPS (lines 8–15). Finally, in lines 15 and 16, the doctor explicitly links the patient's mental illness to his inability to "provide for himself, to survive," thus establishing an assessment that visibly addresses the statutory criteria for commitment.

Many doctors, especially those experienced at testifying in commitment hearings, offer the connection between medical diagnosis and legal charges without prompts.

[4:6]   [Metropolitan Court; J1, DA4, PD2, Dr16, Polly Brown]

1.	DA4:	Based on your opinion of the patient's mental illness, do you
2.		feel that she is capable of providing for her own food, clothes,
3.		and shelter?
4.	Dr16:	I don't believe she could. Polly doesn't have any concept of
5.		handling money. She ran up a two-hundred-dollar water bill
6.		taking baths all day and leaving the water running. She spends
7.		large sums on wine, money she can't really afford. She bought
8.		foolish gifts, things she can't afford to be buying. . . . She said
9.		she was going to live in Dallas, said she had a boyfriend there.
10.		(She was very incoherent about where she would live.) She has
11.		been hospitalized about twenty times since 1966, six times in
12.		the last year. Given her history and diagnosis [bipolar
13.		disorder], I have to say that Polly's mental condition makes her
14.		gravely disabled. Due to her mental illness, she has no way
15.		of supporting, looking after herself, no place to live.
16.		She just ends up back in the hospital.

Here the doctor links documents of mental illness and the inability to provide basic necessities in a fashion that addresses the requirements of commitment law. He also connects the patient's history of recurrent hospitalizations to her inability to provide for herself, suggesting that her frequent readmissions were themselves evidence that she met the criteria for grave disability (lines 10–14). She couldn't provide for herself so the hospital was repeatedly taking over for her (lines 14–16). All of this is accomplished without intervention by the DA, who offered no further questions, implying that he considered the doctor's arguments legally and persuasively adequate. A variant of this sequence appears in extract [3:1], where once again the litany for assembling a visibly warranted recommendation is apparent.

The pattern of first establishing the method and grounds for an assessment, then the psychiatric evaluation or diagnosis itself, and finally the medicolegal assessment and rationale appeared in virtually every case observed. The psychiatrists were prompted to display that they were familiar with the person in question and that they had developed a professional diagnosis out of this familiarity. This diagnosis was then linked to arguments concerning the legal categories of danger or disability. The DA's questioning thus elicited a corpus of evidence that visibly supported the case for commitment, displaying along the way that the argument was grounded in both proper psychiatric methodology and correct understanding of the law.

In every case observed, the testifying psychiatrist argued at this juncture in the proceedings that the patient met the legal criteria for commitment. The doctor's testimony was—except for rare exceptions—the sole basis for the DA's case to commit. While this is the most significant feature of this segment of the proceedings, several important precedents for subsequent testimony are also established in this sequence.

In all cases, the DA addressed the witness as "doctor," while referring to the patient by name or calling him or her "the patient." This referential talk places its objects in membership categories (Sacks 1972) that are subsequently used to interpret, justify, and rationalize testimony and arguments. For example, by establishing the witness as a doctor—first through prior questioning where credentials are displayed, then through the repeated use of the categorization device—and demonstrating that he or she has conscientiously followed a rigorous diagnostic procedure, the DA installs the psychiatrist as a qualified expert and authenticates his or her diagnosis and opinions. The doctor's testimony may be heard as technically warranted and professionally objective. The witness is granted the right to offer psychiatric interpretations that formulate behaviors as symptoms.

In addition, the witness's membership in this category stands as background against which all other testimony—by the doctor and by other witnesses—is heard. The implicit contrast between doctor and patient (or mere civilian) further authorizes the psychiatrist to pass judgment regarding the patient's condition. Chapter 7 discusses how this contrast undermines counterclaims by the patient.

Referring to the subject of this testimony as *patient* has an analogous effect, categorizing the person so that subsequent descriptions of his or her behavior can be heard as symptoms or documents of the mental disorder that led him or her into hospitalization. A similar framing is accomplished when the psychiatrist offers a diagnosis as a global, unequivocal characterization; as in extract [4:4], the *patient is* a "chronic schizophrenic" (line 2)—a distinctive type of person with distinguishing traits. The characterization is offered first, providing a "scheme of interpretation" (Schutz 1970) that can be used to organize and understand subsequent testimony. Lines 5–8 are then offered as motivation for the preceding diagnosis, but they are compelling as documents of mental illness only in light of that diagnosis. The DA has structured the assessment of the patient's mental status so that the general pattern provided by the diagnosis informs the understanding of its symptoms, which can then stand as documents of and warrant for the diagnosis itself.

The process is demonstrated again in example [4:5], where the psychiatrist concludes that the patient is "gravely disabled" (line 5). He infers that this renders the patient unable to function socially, then invokes lack of "social skills" (line 7) as the basis for the grave disability assessment. In this instance, grave disability is invoked as both cause and consequence. These instances of "documentary interpretation" (Garfinkel 1967), then, rely upon the sequential elicitation of interpretive frameworks that afford descriptions the opportunity to reflexively inform their own meaning.

Cross-Examination: Challenging the Psychiatric Assessment

Once a psychiatric assessment has been offered, the DA typically thanks the witness and terminates the direct examination. The PD then cross-examines. This phase of the sequence usually challenges the psychiatric assessment in one (or some combination) of three ways. First, the witness's qualifications as a psychiatric authority might be impugned by questioning his or her training, certification, or experience, especially if these items had not been clearly established in direct examination. This tack was infrequently pursued, and terminated rather quickly if the doctor was able to provide conventional answers.

Alternatively, the PD might challenge the methods the doctor used to produce his or her diagnosis and/or assessment. Most frequently, the PD asks about the doctor's familiarity with the patient, probing further if the doctor indicated that he or she was not the treating physician.[3] In the following case, for example, the PD attempted to show that the testifying doctor was not sufficiently familiar with the patient to make a viable assessment.

[4:7]   [Metropolitan Court; J1, DA6, PD3, Dr17, Mehrangiz Irfani]

1.	PD3:	Is Mrs. Irfani your patient, Dr. Buerer?
2.	Dr17:	I'm on staff at Metro [the state psychiatric hospital], but
3.		she's not my patient, no.
4.	PD3:	Have you interviewed her?
5.	Dr17:	Yes.
6.	PD3:	When was that?
7.	Dr17:	This morning.
8.	PD3:	Here in the courtroom?
9.	Dr17:	That's correct. We didn't have time before the bus [from the
10.		hospital to court] left.

11. PD3: About how long did you speak with her?
12. Dr17: We spoke for about five minutes and it was clear that she was
13. gravely disabled.
14. PD3: So you can make that sort of determination from a five-minute
15. conversation?
16. Dr17: Well from that and by looking at her records and Doctor Maier's
17. recommendations.
18. PD3: Now besides this five-minute chat, have you ever even seen
19. Mrs. Irfani before?
20. Dr17: I don't think so.
21. PD3: Let me ask you, why is it you think she is gravely disabled?
22. Dr17: She is completely disoriented. ((pause to look at patient's
23. hospital chart)) Can't seem to function in her daily life. She
24. gets confused, forgets things, makes wild accusations. She's
25. been delusional. ((pause to look at chart)) She says that her
26. husband is trying to get her to sleep with other men.
27. PD3: Is that true? Have you asked her husband?
28. Dr17: From my understanding of Iranian customs, sleeping with someone
29. you're not married to is strictly prohibited. She says that her
30. husband is making her do all sorts of things. She says he's
31. watching her through a TV camera.
32. PD3: But have you asked him about this doctor, talked to the husband?
33. Dr17: No I haven't been in touch with him.

Here, the PD challenged the doctor's assessment methods by implying that his contact with the patient was brief and perfunctory. In addition, the PD also questioned the doctor's acceptance of the husband's claims about his wife without question or corroboration. Later, in his summation, the PD argued that Dr. Buerer was so unfamiliar with the case and the persons involved that the doctor's conclusions were "unfounded." He further argued that the doctor "hardly spoke with my client," and his assessment was "based on accusations by a husband who was never even consulted. . . . Why should we take his word over hers?"

A third means of challenging the psychiatric assessment focused on the doctor's medicolegal opinion. While PDs routinely questioned doctors' qualifications and assessment procedures, they never directly challenged their psychiatric *diagnoses*. As a consequence, all cases proceeded with the understanding that the patient was mentally ill. But questions were often raised concerning the way determinations of danger or grave disability were assembled and linked to the patient's illnesses. This approach was perhaps the most common strategy for challenging recommendations to commit, as PDs probed the reasoning that psychiatrists offered for their assessments, exploring the ways that reports of the patient's condition and behavior were linked to both the psychiatric diagnosis and the commitment recommendation.

Questioning sequences might take several forms. One tack was to challenge the factual bases for the doctors' conclusions. PDs might question doctors' judgments about what was treated as truth, misinformation, delusion, hallucination, and the like. Recall, for example, that the psychiatrist in extract [4:6] argued that Polly Brown was financially irresponsible, citing the fact that she incurred phenomenal water bills by bathing excessively. During cross-examination, the PD in the case challenged this portion of the testimony.

[4:8]   [Metropolitan Court; J1, DA4, PD2, Dr16, Polly Brown]

1.	PD2:	Where is Ms. Brown currently living?
2.	Dr16:	Presently she lives with her mother and sister.
3.	PD2:	Did you ever see that water bill you mentioned?
4.	Dr16:	No.
5.	PD2:	Does she have a separate meter from the rest of the family?
6.	Dr16:	I don't know about that.
7.	PD2:	Was this a monthly bill? How long was this bill for?
8.	Dr16:	Her mother said it was for one month.
9.	PD2:	Now, how did her mother determine that it was her [Polly] that
10.		ran up this bill?
11.	Dr16:	I don't know. The mother just said // she did.
12.	J1:	((breaking in)) How would she know that?
13.	PD2:	Your honor I'm just trying to establish the fact that there were
14.		several people in the household and if a lot of water was being
15.		used, the others must have been using some of it and it's not
16.		proven that Ms. Brown was responsible for this bill.
17.	J1:	You've made your point, Mr. Webster. Let's continue.

Here, the PD questioned the doctor's conclusion that Ms. Brown had incurred the water bill, attempting to undermine the most vivid item of anecdotal evidence supporting the contention that Brown was gravely disabled. As was often the case, the doctor used examples of bizarre conduct to corroborate his allegations. Because claims were frequently documented anecdotally, with little attempt to argue the relative frequencies of "normal" versus "abnormal" or "problematic" behavior, discrediting or negating a single example might serve to undercut an entire argument. Of course, the psychiatric testimony was necessarily selective, but relying upon anecdotal arguments often left it vulnerable to this sort of attack.

An alternative strategy used to contest medicolegal assessments involved questioning the psychiatric witness's judgment regarding the application of the legal categories of danger or disability to the case at hand. In Gloria Madden's hearing, for example, the doctor testified that Ms. Madden was a danger to others, citing reports that she had been wandering in traffic with a knife, threatening to harm bystanders, then turning on the police when they arrived on the scene. During cross-examination, the PD questioned the doctor's conclusion.

[4:9] [Metropolitan Court; J1, DA2, PD1, Dr9, Gloria Madden]

1.	PD1:	Your decision is that Gloria is dangerous to others, correct?
2.	Dr9:	That's my opinion.
3.	PD1:	Has she had any fights on the ward since she's been
4.		hospitalized?
5.	Dr9:	No.
6.	PD1:	Has she been verbally abusive of other patients or the staff?
7.	Dr9:	No.
8.	PD1:	Has she hurt anyone, either before she was arrested or after
9.		she's been on the ward?
10.	Dr9:	Not to my knowledge.
11.	PD1:	Has she tried to obtain any sort of weapon, secret kitchen
12.		utensils, things like that?
13.	Dr9:	Not that I know of.
14.		((silence five seconds))
15.	PD1:	Now, doctor, has Gloria been hospitalized before?

Later, the PD summarized his argument, stating that there was no direct evidence that Ms. Madden had ever hurt anyone—that she never so much as threatened a dangerous act while under observation.[4]

Rather than disputing the facts of the case at hand as the doctor presented them, the PD here attempted to elicit an alternative set of facts that could later be cited as grounds for questioning the doctor's judgment that the patient was a danger to others. In this particular instance, the questioning was organized to reveal a set of observations about the patient that was inconsistent with the doctor's ultimate assessment. The inconsistency was then invoked to argue that the assessment was flawed. Frequently, PDs attempted to establish discrepancies between the problematic conduct cited in doctors' testimony and behavior that the doctors had witnessed in the hospital (but not mentioned). This provided the basis for arguing either that the doctor's judgment of the patient's condition was erroneous or that the initial assessment might have been valid, but the patient had sufficiently improved while hospitalized so that release was now appropriate.

This strategy of contradicting the doctor's previously stated medicolegal assessment was an especially prevalent tactic in cases where grave disability was charged. PDs routinely acknowledged the validity of the doctors' diagnoses but asked questions to explore the relationship between a patient's mental illness and his or her ability to provide food, clothing, and shelter. The following case illustrates a straightforward attempt to demonstrate that mental illness alone did not qualify a patient for commitment. Under direct examination, Dr. Fischer had testified that Regina Farmer was gravely disabled because her mental disturbance (PCP psychosis combined with bipolar disorder) had rendered her unable to provide for food, clothing, and shelter (see Appendix 2). In an extended cross-examination, the PD repeatedly attempted to dissolve the connection between Ms. Farmer's mental problems and the practical disabilities that comprise grave disability.

[4:10]   [Metropolitan Court; J2, DA1, PD3, Dr2, Regina Farmer]

1.	PD3:	In addition to her problem with PCP, is this woman mentally ill?
2.		((silence)) Is this problem a serious mental illness?
3.	Dr2:	That's a hard question. In my opinion she also has a bipolar
4.		disorder.
5.	PD3:	Is PCP psychosis an LPS illness, a mental illness? Is it a
6.		serious problem?
7.	Dr2:	Yes combined with the bipolar disorder, it's a very serious
8.		disorder uh illness.
9.	PD3:	So you're convinced that Ms. Farmer is gravely disabled.
10.	Dr2:	That's right.
11.	PD3:	OK, now is the patient oriented to time and place?
12.	Dr2:	Yes.
13.	PD3:	Where has she been living?
14.	Dr2:	She's been living with her grandmother.
15.	PD3:	Does she know her grandmother's phone number?
16.	Dr2:	I think so.
17.	PD3:	Does she know her relatives' names?
18.	Dr2:	Yes.
19.	PD3:	Is she well enough to get home from here by herself?
20.	Dr2:	I suppose so.
21.	PD3:	Can she ride the bus?
22.	Dr2:	Yes.
23.	PD3:	Does she feed and dress herself in the hospital?
24.	Dr2:	As far as I know.
25.	PD3:	Does she understand that it's important to take care of herself,
26.		eat regularly, have a place to stay?
27.	Dr2:	She seems to.
28.	PD3:	Would she go get something to eat if she were hungry?
29.	Dr2:	Yes.
30.	PD3:	So she could take herself down to McDonalds for lunch by
31.		herself?
32.	Dr2:	Yes, I suppose.

33.	J2:	Now I'm not so sure that McDonalds really qualifies as food,
34.		does it Mr. Patrick. [general laughter in courtroom]
35.	PD3:	((laughs)) Arguably. ((silence)) Now doctor, would you say that
36.		Ms.Farmer's symptoms are abating?
37.	Dr2:	Yes, slightly.
38.	PD3:	And why is it, then that she is unable to provide for her own
39.		food, clothing, and shelter?
40.	Dr2:	She's very confused, delusional, assaultive, threatening. These
41.		things, these behaviors interfere with interpersonal
42.		transactions. She functions very poorly and has poor
43.		reality contact //
44.	PD3:	((breaking in)) What, what delusions has she displayed?
45.	Dr2:	Only the one about being a TV star.
46.	PD3:	But she doesn't have delusions that have anything to do with
47.		food, clothing, or shelter? ((silence)) She isn't afraid of food
48.		for instance?
49.	Dr2:	No, she just has very bad judgment, very confused.
50.	PD3:	That's all, Dr. Fischer. Thank you.

Later, in his summation, the PD argued that his client should not be hospitalized "simply on the basis of being mentally ill," and referred to the doctor's answers to the above series of questions as evidence that Ms. Farmer's mental illness did not prevent her from providing for her basic necessities, as the doctor had claimed.

Viewed holistically, this extract reveals the PD's attempt to separate Ms. Farmer's mental illness from her ability to provide food, clothing, and shelter. Also embedded in the exchange is a strategy for discrediting the doctor's testimony by asking questions ostensibly designed to clarify matters, but doing so in a way that implies that the doctor's opinion was inconsistent or open to doubt. The PD begins by implicitly questioning the doctor's diagnosis, questioning the assertion that Ms. Farmer's mental problem was a "serious mental illness" (lines 1–27). When the doctor equivocates (line 3), the PD repeats his question (line 5–6). The doctor reasserts that the problem is indeed a serious illness (line 7–8), leading the PD to assume an alternative line of questioning (but note that the doctor labels the problem a serious *illness* only as a correction of his initial use of *disorder* to characterize the problem).

This new line focuses on the practical aspects of grave disability, each question designed to elicit a piece of information that might belie the assertion that Ms. Farmer could not provide for her basic needs. Even the discussion of Ms. Farmer's delusions is brought back to the issue of their relevance to her ability to provide food, clothing, and shelter. The sequence of questions provides a framework for displaying inconsistencies between the doctor's general assessment and his appraisals of discrete instances of Ms. Farmer's behavior. After the doctor confirms his claim that Ms. Farmer is gravely disabled (line 10), for example, the PD elicits ten consecutive assessments by the doctor (lines 11–32) that fail to support—indeed they arguably contradict—the judgment of grave disability.

In this exchange, the PD's questioning produced a series of implicit contrasts that have damaging implications for the witness's medicolegal conclusion. Drew (1985) argues that "contrast devices" like this are commonly used as rhetorical resources in legal as well as nonlegal settings. Their recurrent use and forcefulness, he suggests, are particularly evident in courtroom cross-examination, and this is clearly true in commitment hearings. Extract [4:9] further illustrates the practice. In this instance, the PD invites the psychiatrist to reaffirm that the patient is dangerous to others (lines 1–2) and then generates a series of questions and answers that contradict this assertion. The inconsistency is apparent.

Note, however, that it is not directly mentioned by the PD. Nor is the witness asked to account for the contradiction. As in extracts [4:9] and [4:10], damaging disjunctures between aspects of the psychiatric assessments are produced, but they are left as unresolved puzzles as the line of questioning is terminated. Again, this is a common cross-examination device (Drew 1985) used to damage witnesses' testimony. Counsel generates the puzzle, then denies the witness the opportunity to provide explanations or account for the apparent incongruities. The inferences that might be suggested are left implicit, inviting hearers, most specifically the judge, to draw for themselves the damaging implications that emerge from discrepant testimony. Indeed, PDs often provide the opportunity to note and reflect upon the implications that may be drawn from the contrasts by pausing before moving to new lines of questioning. In extract [4:9], for instance, the PD permits a five-second silence to develop after his questioning sequence (line 14), allowing hearers to contemplate the series of responses that seem to contradict the doctor's claim that the patient was dangerous. The silence tacitly exploits the contrasts, while the subsequent move to a new line of questioning (line 15) denies the witness the opportunity to explain the discrepancies. Even though contradictions are made visible, they are typically not mentioned until PDs' closing summations. They may be resurrected as a resource for refuting the psychiatric testimony at a juncture where there is typically little chance for the DA or psychiatrist to refute or explain them away.

Before the psychiatrist is excused (to reoccupy a seat in the courtroom gallery), the judge often asks questions of his own. Typically, he seeks to clarify answers to previous questions, especially those regarding the doctor's rationale for his or her assessment. Judges also ask questions regarding how patients have been doing while hospitalized, inquiring into the doctors' opinions regarding the advisability of placing the patient in various community treatment and support programs. While judges' questions are most often raised at the end of cross-examination, they might be interjected at any time. Sometimes they are not raised at all.

After the PD concludes cross-examination and the judge has his opportunity to question, the PD is routinely asked if he or she is going to call any witnesses. This presupposes that the DA has no further witnesses, which is almost always the case. In those instances, the DA interrupted to indicate that there were more witnesses to be heard. The request was always granted, and the additional witness—usually a family member of the patient—testified.

Organizing the Patient's Rebuttal

Since the burden of proof in commitment hearings lies with the state, PDs were not required to make a case for their patients'release. The PD, however, called a witness—the patient—in over 90 percent of the cases I observed. PDs explained that they declined to let the patient testify only when they were certain that he or she would be unable to testify coherently and rationally. They believed that judges assumed that a failure to testify indicated that the patient was too deranged to manage consequential social interactions. Judges confirmed this belief; they felt that a patient who did not testify must be so disturbed that the PD knew the patient was a liability to the case. Consequently, PDs encouraged their clients to testify, even if they suspected that their clients would "act crazy."[5]

Direct Examination: Rebutting Prior Testimony

The patient was the sole witness called by PDs in all cases observed in Metropolitan Court, and in all but one of the other proceedings observed. The PD's questions for the patient were typically simple and straightforward—often answerable in single words or sentences. Elaborations were generally discouraged. The PD's inquiries usually related to lines of questioning opened in the direct examination of the psychiatric witness. Some sequences sought to produce sets of facts—as recounted from the patient's point of view—that might rival those reported by the doctor. Other sequences attempted to established alternative interpretations of facts previously noted. In the case involving

Polly Brown (extracts [4:6] and [4:8]; Appendix 1), for example, the psychiatrist had testified that, among other things, Ms. Brown was financially irresponsible and had incurred a two-hundred-dollar water bill by bathing excessively. Moreover, the doctor contended that Ms. Brown had no place to live. The PD used Ms. Brown's appearance on the witness stand as an opportunity to present the patient's version of these circumstances.

[4:11]   [Metropolitan Court; J1, DA4, PD2, Dr16, Polly Brown]

1.	PD2:	If the judge releases you, Polly, where will you go?
2.	PB:	I'll go with my children. We'll live at my mother's house.
3.	PD2:	Is that OK with her?
4.	PB:	Of course. She's my mother, my family. She won't kick me out
5.		// for a little fussin.
6.	PD2:	((breaking in)) How long have you lived with your mother?
7.	PB:	I've been there approximately three years.
8.	PD2:	Have you ever lived in Dallas?
9.	PB:	I spent the whole summer there.
10.	PD2:	Did you say that you'd move to Dallas if you got out of Metro?
11.	PB:	I'm hoping to go to Dallas someday. Not now. I want to get
12.		away from here eventually. The state of California is crippling
13.		my mind. But I'm not crazy. // I'm fine. I'm intelligent.
14.		I'll go wherever I want.
15.	PD2:	((breaking in)) But you'll go to your mother's first.
16.	PB:	Of course.
17.	PD2:	Is it true that your mother said she doesn't want you to stay
18.		with her any more?
19.	PB:	That's a lie. She said she would take me. She can't come
20.		today, but a friend of mine will pick me up and take me home.
21.		(PD asks several questions regarding Ms. Brown's ability to
22.		provide for her food, clothing, and shelter. Ms. Brown indicates
23.		that she can provide these things.)
24.	PD2:	Are you responsible for a two-hundred-dollar water bill, Polly?
25.	PB:	That's ridiculous. There ain't no two-hundred-dollar bill.
26.	PD2:	Then why did the doctor mention it?
27.	PB:	I don't know. Maybe my mama said so and got confused.

While the sequence is not a point-by-point rebuttal of the doctor's prior testimony, it is designed to elicit alternative depictions of events and circumstances that the doctor had previously characterized. For example, the PD selected three issues that had previously been raised in the psychiatric testimony as illustrations of Ms. Brown's troubles (the two-hundred-dollar water bill, lack of a reasonable place to live, and ability to provide food, clothing, and shelter). His questions let Ms.

Brown present her versions of the matters in question, producing depictions that were subsequently incorporated into the PD's argument that the psychiatrist had incorrectly understood Ms. Brown's circumstances and behavior.

The PD's questions for the patient also addressed the legal requirements for commitment—danger and disability. A common sequence in grave disability cases, for example, moves directly to the patient's appraisal of his or her ability to provide basic necessities. In the following case, where grave disability had been charged, the patient was thoroughly questioned regarding matters pertaining to shelter, nourishment, money, and other practical concerns.

[4:12]   [Metropolitan Court; J1, DA5, PD4, Dr4, Jason Andro]

1.	PD4:	Mr. Andro, do you want to get out of the hospital?
2.	JA:	Yes ma'am.
3.	PD4:	Can you take care of yourself?
4.	JA:	Yes ma'am.
5.	PD4:	Where would you stay?
6.	JA:	With my parents. Or maybe at a friend's house.
7.	PD4:	Which friend?
8.	JA:	I have a couple in mind. // They've done it before.
9.	PD4:	((breaking in)) Have you been employed?
10.	JA:	Yes, I've done all types of food preparation. You know, working
11.		in restaurants.
12.	PD4:	If you had some money, say four hundred dollars, could you tell
13.		us how you would use it to take care of yourself?
14.	JA:	The first thing I would do would be to buy a car // so I
15.	J1:	((breaking in)) What? Why a car?
16.	JA:	I'd get a car to travel around to find a job.
17.	PD4:	OK now. If you had some money, how much would you spend on
18.		rent?
19.	JA:	Nothing if I'm at home. I suppose I should give something if
20.		I crash with a friend though.
21.	PD4:	What about meals?
22.	JA:	I can fix anything. I learned in the restaurants.
23.	PD4:	Would you eat regularly?
24.	JA:	Yes ma'am.
25.	PD4:	Would you take your medications if you were released?
26.	JA:	I guess. ((silence)) Yes ma'am, I'll take it.
27.	PD4:	Will you go to an outpatient program?
28.	JA:	Yes, I've done that before.
29.	PD4:	Do you feel like you've improved since you've been in the
30.		hospital?
31.	JA:	Yes ma'am. One hundred percent // I'm a new man.

Sequences like [4:12] implicitly challenge doctors' medicolegal assessments by displaying the patient's ability to obtain basic necessities, providing an alternative to the doctor's grave disability assessment. The approach avoids direct challenges to the doctor's diagnosis or psychiatric expertise per se. Instead, the PD implicitly questions the doctor's judgment of the patient's routine and mundane functioning, allowing the patient to speak for him- or herself. Related lines of questioning often extend to the issues of the patient's assessment of his or her own condition, as well as his or her willingness to comply with outpatient treatment and medication regimes—again matters where professional expertise may be countered by the patient's own claims.

Cross-Examination: Challenging the Patient's Version

At the completion of the patient's direct testimony, the DA typically (although not invariably) cross-examined. Frequently, the cross-examination resumed lines of questioning raised during direct examination, providing the opportunity for elaboration of answers previously given. These sequences often included pointed and dubious inquiries into prior answers. In a hearing involving Rachel Dunstan, for example, the PD had asked the patient a series of brief questions about how she would provide for her food, clothing, and shelter. The questions were nearly all answerable in a single word or phrase (e.g., Would you eat if you got hungry? Will you stay at your mother's house? How will you support yourself?). Ms. Dunstan answered all questions very briefly and straightforwardly, indicating that she would be able to provide for herself. The cross-examination reopened these issues.

[4:13]   [Eastern Court; J1, DA2, PD1, Dr2, Rachel Dunstan]

1.	DA2:	You said that you will be able to take care of yourself if
2.		you're discharged. Are you sure that you can stay with your
3.		mother?
4.	RD:	I always have.
5.	DA2:	But what about all the things you said to her. Are you going to
6.		be able to keep from yelling at her again?
7.	RD:	I didn't say any such thing.
8.	DA2:	But she says you did, and she won't put up with it. What if it
9.		starts again and she makes you leave?
10.	RD:	I'll find a place.
11.	DA2:	But you don't have any place in mind?
12.	RD:	Not right now.
13.	DA2:	And what if you can't get your job back? [RD had claimed that

14.   she would resume her job as a janitor in an office building.]
15.   RD: I'll get the job. I've worked there before.
16.   DA2: But you were never hospitalized on the job before.
17.   RD: It won't matter. Mr. Stevens [the boss] likes me.
18.   DA2: But he might have filled your job. What if you can't get it
19.   back?
20.   RD: I don't know about that.
21.   DA2: Well how will you support yourself then?
22.   RD: I'll manage. I can work for someone else.

Here, the DA reformulated prior questions about Ms. Dunstan's projected living circumstances and her anticipated job, declining to accept Ms. Dunstan's responses without elaboration. He posed hypothetical complications to the scenarios that Ms. Dunstan previously described, asking her to speculate about possible complicating contingencies that he implied were likely to arise. Such sequences were used to address the patient's command of the practical circumstances of his or her life—as did questions during direct examination—but within in an environment of skepticism. Whereas PDs typically solicited answers that could briefly and directly confirm the patient's ability to provide food, clothing, and shelter, DAs' cross-examinations implied considerable doubt about prior claims. Consider the difference, for example, between the way the PD established Rachel Dunstan's ability to provide for food, clothing, and shelter and the technique used by the DA to challenge Dunstan's initial claim. The PD asked Ms. Dunstan very straightforwardly: "If they let you go, can you provide for your own food, clothes, and a place to live, Rachel?" Ms. Dunstan's response was a simple "Yes." Contrast this with the sequence of questions in extract [4:13] in which the DA broke the question into components, then phrased a series of questions so that each cast doubt on Ms. Dunstan's prior answers (see [4:13], lines 1–3, 5–6, 8–9, 11, 13–14, 18–19).

In addition, cross-examinations often encouraged patients to elaborate prior answers, seeking responses that might reveal greater uncertainty than previously indicated. While direct examination generally posed the least complicated scenarios that the patient might encounter, cross-examination complicated the situations in ways that were likely to entice equivocal responses or confusion. Note, for example, the way the DA in extract [4:13] reformulated postrelease scenarios to pose hypothetically complicated circumstances to which he then asked the patient to respond.

DAs also employed an alternative line of questioning that required patients to respond to matters not previously mentioned or emphasized. Frequently, these inquiries raised new issues regarding the provision of basic necessities that the patient may have glossed over or refrained from mentioning in prior testimony. They also introduced new factors that might bear upon the case, either in terms of facts regarding the provision of basic necessities, or regarding the patient's condition more generally. For example, DAs questioned patients about behaviors noted in the patients' psychiatric records that had not been mentioned during psychiatric testimony, as in the case involving Jason Andro (also shown in extract [4:12] and Appendix 3).

[4:14]   [Metropolitan Court; J1, DA5, PD4, Dr4, Jason Andro]

1.	DA5:	Is it true that you heard from your brother before you left
2.		Tucson telling you to come to California?
3.	JA:	Yeah I did.
4.	DA5:	And tell us how you heard from your brother?
5.	JA:	A thing called love. I heard through a thing called love, you
6.		know.
7.	DA5:	A thing called love?
8.	JA:	Yeah you all know what that is.
9.	DA5:	I suppose. When you were admitted to the hospital were you
10.		delusional?
11.	JA:	Yes ma'am, but I'm not now.
12.	DA5:	The doctor says you've been calling yourself Hercules. Why?
13.	JA:	Look at me. I look like Hercules don't I? I am the one.
14.	DA5:	What does that mean?
15.	JA:	You know, the one. The powerful one. You know who I am.
16.	DA5:	Oh?
		(Several questions and answers intervene.)
17.	DA5:	Haven't you said that your brother is Jesus Christ?
18.	JA:	Yes I think so. Ever since he was born I could see he was
19.		Christ. I guess I saw this when I was about eighteen. About
20.		four years ago.
21.	DA5:	Are you sure?
22.	JA:	As sure as I can be.
23.	DA5:	But didn't you also say that your mother was the devil?
24.	JA:	Yes. I've seen it in her eyes.
25.		((silence))
26.	JA:	It's very difficult with her. Sometimes I find it hard to live
27.		at home.
28.	DA5:	Do you want to live at home now?
29.	JA:	Yes I do. I can do it because I have the power.
30.	DA5:	The power?
31.	JA:	That's right, the power. You know what I mean.
32.	DA5:	That's all Mr. Andro.

In this sequence, the DA asked Mr. Andro about four different matters that his medical record apparently noted but that had not been previously mentioned in this hearing (i.e., how he heard from his brother, calling himself Hercules, calling his brother Jesus Christ, and calling his mother the devil). Such sequences illustrate medical claims about the patient or promote firsthand displays of his or her symptoms. DAs report that evidence of symptomatology is not generated to confirm psychiatric diagnoses; rather they claim it is used to display the patient's inability to manage consequential aspects of his or her daily life. Symptomatic displays may also serve as background against which patients' claims can be evaluated. By inducing "crazy" or "delusional" talk, DAs can discredit other claims patients might make in their own defense.[6]

In sum, cross-examination generally involved questions whose answers held the potential to undermine patients' rebuttals of the charges lodged against them. DAs formulated series of questions that provided multiple opportunities for patients to discredit their own claims. They manipulated the sequential environment of questions and answers so as require more elaborate, complicated answers than those demanded by PDs. Whereas PDs used contrast devices to display inconsistencies within psychiatrists' testimony, DAs frequently attempted to produce visible disjunctures between what the doctors reported about patients and the patients' claims about those same matters. Given the prevailing assumptions that psychiatrists are knowledgeable expert witnesses and that patients are mentally ill, DAs felt that discrepancies were likely to be interpreted as evidence of faulty perceptions or reports by the patients. Thus, contradictions between doctor and patient were viewed as probative of claims that the patient was indeed out of touch with his or her conditions and/or circumstances.

While DAs attempted to produce discrepancies between patients' claims and "more reliable" testimony, they did much less contextualizing work than PDs, treating damaging testimony by patients as if it were "obvious." DAs were more likely, for example, to simply let patients' claims "speak for themselves." Testimony that DAs figured was evidence of psychiatric disorder or interactional incompetence was not juxtaposed with normal or competent examples. Instead, DAs relied on the unspoken assumption that severe problems were clearly visible to competent members of the courtroom. Later, however, in their summations DAs would cite disturbances and disorders, treating them as accepted matters of fact.

Attorneys' Comments and Summations

Before the patient was excused from the witness stand, the judge often asked questions to elaborate and clarify issues that might have been raised (see Appendix 2, for example). This did not happen in every case, nor was there a discernible pattern to the questions that might be raised. Finally, after the patient's testimony, the PD and the DA were given an opportunity to comment upon aspects of the case and to summarize their arguments. It was not uncommon, however, for one or both attorneys to decline and offer instead to simply "submit it." In those instances where summations were forthcoming, the arguments typically addressed the statutory requirements for commitment in very direct fashion, often in the literal language of the statutes. A PD might simply argue, for example, that "We contend there has been insufficient evidence produced to establish Mr. Stankowitz's grave disability." Conversely, DAs often confined their summations to brief statements like "Mr. Manuel clearly meets the criteria under LPS. The doctor has diagnosed him as seriously ill and has testified that he cannot provide for his food, clothing, and shelter."

Many summations, especially the PDs', were somewhat more elaborate. The elaborations typically articulated in greater detail a set of reasons why the circumstances of the case at hand failed to meet the statutory requirements for commitment. Most frequently, these arguments projected the law onto the case at hand, noting that symptoms of mental illness were not sufficient grounds for involuntary hospitalization. Regina Farmer's case (see extract [4:10] and Appendix 2) is exemplary in this regard.

[4:15]   [Metropolitan Court; J2, DA1, PD3, Dr2, Regina Farmer]

PD3:

> We just don't think Ms. Farmer is gravely disabled your honor. Under LPS, involuntary hospitalization should not detain a person simply on the basis of being mentally ill. A person can be hospitalized only if he can't provide for his own food, clothes, and shelter. (I understand the doctor's position and why he thinks the patient is mentally ill. I won't argue about the diagnosis.) But the symptoms are receding. And more important, they don't interfere with Ms. Farmer's providing for her own food, clothes, and shelter. If her delusions dealt with food, clothes, and shelter, I'd be concerned, but even if she can't stay with her mother or grandmother, she can take care of herself. (She can stay with other relatives. There are several in the area.) Just because she's on thin ice with her family is no reason to commit her. We have lots of people go through here who are on thin ice with their families, but that's not the basis on which you judge them. (My client does not meet the criteria for LPS.)

While this summation is more elaborate, detailed, and systematic than most, it models PDs' efforts to display (1) the requirements of the law, (2) the circumstances of the case at hand, and (3) the ways that the case fails to meet the legal requirements. More typically, PDs more concisely articulated a limited set of ways in which their clients failed to meet legal criteria. The facts of the case might be disputed and the doctors medicolegal assessment challenged. The diagnoses, however, were never directly questioned as the arguments focused on the practical rather than the medical side of the assessment.

DAs were less likely than PDs to formally summarize their cases. When they did, they were typically less elaborate. Like PDs, they offered linkages between legal criteria and the circumstances of the case at hand. The following summation, from the case involving Jason Andro (also see Appendix 3), displays the way DAs might do this.

[4:16] [Metropolitan Court; J1, DA5, PD4, Dr4, Jason Andro]

DA5:

> Dr. Chin indicates that Mr. Andro is delusional and this will interfere with carrying out his day-to-day efforts to provide for himself. (He has no income and no one eager to support him. He quit a job in order to look for another one in a time of a bad economy, and that shows very poor judgment. He says he wants to work in a job that he's never done before. He has no place to stay and no prospects for finding one. He will have trouble providing for his food, clothes, and shelter even if he does manage to move in with someone.) A man his age should be able to support himself and he can't. His mental illness makes him unemployable. It makes him unable to take care of himself. People who can take care of themselves don't say and do the kind of things he does. He seems to meet every angle of LPS.

Resolution

Involuntary commitment hearings conclude with some form of resolution to the case at hand. Most frequently, this involves the judge's decision to commit or release the patient, accompanied by a brief explanation. Typically, these accounts orient to the statutory requirements for commitment in the same ways as the attorneys' summations, as in the following example.

[4:17] [Metropolitan Court; J1, DA4, PD1, Dr18, Peter Elias]

J1:

> I don't think the court is as convinced as Mr. Black [the PD] that this patient should be released. I'm finding Mr. Elias gravely disabled and unable to provide food, clothing, and shelter. There's no indication of any place to go here, and these symptoms are not sufficiently diminished for him to take care of himself. I don't see him being responsible for getting all the things he needs, and he doesn't have anyone who can do it for him.

In this instance, the judge indicated that he found the patient gravely disabled because he was unable to provide food, clothing, and shelter, then elaborated why he thought this to be the case. Release could be explained in a similar fashion.

[4:18] [Metropolitan Court; J2, DA2, PD5, Dr1, Albert Marco]

J2:

> I'm not convinced of grave disability here, so I'll grant the writ. Mr. Marco says he'll return to the board and care home and stay in the program. As long as he's there, he should be taken care of, so his food, clothing, and shelter are not in jeopardy.

Not all cases ended in such clear-cut, unilateral decisions. Occasionally, the judge might render a decision that was contingent upon some response or concession by the patient, granting release only if the patient agreed to specific demands. It was not uncommon for Metropolitan Court judges to grant release "as soon as someone shows up to claim him [or her]," indicating that the patient had to leave the court in the company of the person the patient claimed he or she would live with and/or be responsible to. If this could not be arranged, the patient was returned to the hospital. Release might also be granted on conditions of taking up residence in a board and care home, enrolling in community-based treatment programs, or voluntarily submitting to inpatient psychiatric treatment.

Similarly, a judge might uphold the involuntary commitment, but suggest that if specified criteria were met, he would reconsider his decision. In a case involving a Vietnam era army veteran, for example, the judge denied the writ on the grounds of grave disability but suggested that the PD and doctor consult with a county social worker regarding the possibility of obtaining veterans' benefits and treatment at the local VA hospital. The judge then asked the patient if he would go into the VA hospital if he was released from the state hospital. When the patient agreed, the judge concluded: "OK, then, let's work this out. If we can get Mr. Walton into the VA, I may be able to reassess my ruling."

In this instance, and others like it, a legal decision was rendered, but perhaps more importantly, the judge mediated an alternative resolution that was satisfactory to the involved parties. While such outcomes were infrequent, occasionally the judge was able to convince a patient to drop his or her writ application if certain conditions of treatment were met (e.g., termination of certain medications, visitation privileges extended), or if the doctor would agree to recommend release upon completion of some phase of the treatment regime but sooner than the maximum term of hospitalization. Commitment hearings thus concluded with binding legal decisions, some of these representing mediated or negotiated resolutions that were substantially different from simple commitment or release.

Finally, judges often marked the termination of a hearing by initiating a final exchange with the patient. Sometimes it was words of explanation directed to a patient being returned to the hospital. For example, one judge explained, "Mr. Feingold, this will be what's best for you. You'll be with doctors who care very much about you and are trying to help you." Occasions when release was granted were often punctuated with admonitions to the now-free person to do his or her best to stay out of the hospital in the future. In either case, the judge always had the final word, which frequently amounted to "I'm doing what I think is best for you."

Interpretive Issues for Involuntary Commitment

The interrogatory sequence provides a structure for articulating the issues that constitute commitment hearings as medically informed legal proceedings. The sequence ensures that each case includes a psychiatric assessment and charges of danger or grave disability, an opportunity to rebut those charges, and a resolution to the case. Whereas the sequence is present in some form in all cases, its subsequences are diverse and somewhat unsystematic. Questioning formats vary from case to case, attorney to attorney. Assessments and rebuttals are similarly unsystematic; while always present, they are not formulaic. Claims are illustrated and warranted anecdotally, using examples drawn opportunistically from those that may be available. Assertions supported by examples, however, are more likely to be challenged by refuting or denying the examples than by challenging the logic or substance of the arguments. Arguments thus take on a rather piecemeal character that may be challenged in a similarly unsystematic fashion.

Central to all commitment hearings, however, are three interpretive projects that provide the visible bases for warranted judicial decisions: (1) displaying people, (2) depicting circumstances, and (3) making "justice" and "legality" visible.

Displaying People

Legal proceedings rely on descriptions of persons to justify or rationalize arguments and decisions (Maynard 1984). Assigning persons to descriptive categories (e.g., mentally ill, sane, male, female) distinguishes individuals from one another for the purpose of deciding, in the case of commitment hearings, who should be confined and treated and who should be sent out of the courtroom into a relatively "normal" existence. Such categorization practices do more than report on a putative reality; they constitute that reality for the practical purpose at hand. The resolution of a case, then, often amounts to a judicial decision about the descriptive authenticity of alternative depictions.

Portraying personal characteristics and types is not confined to psychiatric diagnoses, although these are among the most important. Commitment hearings also serve as an arena for claims-making about what is normal, expectable, reasonable behavior as well as an opportunity for displaying firsthand the interactional "competence" and "incompetence" of persons whose commitment is sought. The interactional organization of displays of competence is discussed in greater detail in Chapter 5, while Chapter 8 further examines practices of constitutive person description.

Depicting Circumstance

Participants' orientations to the practical aspects of commitment laws also require them to consider a variety of situational contingencies. Arguments, claims, and assessments are frequently justified by reference to the social and material circumstances confronting patients seeking release. Descriptions of patients' conduct and activities, and projections of their future behavior, often incorporate elaborate depictions of settings and contingent scenarios that may be relevant to the issues at hand. Grave disability arguments, for example, often expand to concerns for how a patient conducts him- or herself in the environments he or she will encounter in everyday life outside the hospital. Chapters 6, 7, and 8 analyze some of the ways that depictions of patients' living circumstances are incorporated into commitment arguments.

Doing "Legality" and "Justice"

Commitment hearings must also show that the law has guided the proceedings. Indeed, Warren (1982) notes that a major function of commitment hearings in Metropolitan Court is visibly demonstrating a coherence between the decision-making process and the mandates of the law so that justice is "seen to be done." The interrogatory sequence provides a structure of routine opportunities to display that justice is being done—that is, that laws and procedures are followed to produce fair and humane rulings. This is perhaps most obvious on the numerous occasions that courtroom questions and arguments are articulated in the language of commitment statutes, as well as through ritual demonstration of adherence to procedural rules specifying the temporal and sequential order of conversation. Speakers provided frequent and observable *legal* warrants for their questions and claims, thus documenting and making plainly visible that their conduct was responsive and responsible to the law.[7] Put differently, the law is used as a rhetorical resource, providing legitimation for arguments by incorporating legal principles and reasoning.

While procedural issues are not raised as commonly as in most criminal or civil courtrooms (e.g., procedural objections are uncommon), explicit reference to legal constraints on talk nonetheless distinguishes commitment hearings from scenes of ordinary conversation. Add to this other signals of the legal process being upheld—like the ritual use of ceremonial forms of address (e.g., "Your Honor" for the judge), the "swearing in" of each witness, and official record keeping—and the extent to which discourse practices produce a sense of legal order is apparent.

In addition, the interrogation sequence invites each concerned party to argue his or her case; failures to do so are noted, and explicit encouragement is often forthcoming. The sequence also invites the articulation of explanations and warrants for competing arguments, making it clear that fair consideration was given to all claims. The structure of commitment hearings is thus implicated in both the production of the claims, facts, and warrants upon which judicial decisions are based, and in "doing justice" so that the procedural fairness and legality of the proceedings are clearly evident.

* * * * *

Much of the hearing sequence is devoted to establishing the "competence" of the persons seeking release. Hearing participants constitute documents of mental illness, interactional adequacy, and functional disabilities through exchanges of questions and answers. Chapter 5 examines the interactional practices implicated in the production of signs of patients' interactional competence and incompetence.

Notes

1. The conversational data presented here are reproduced from verbatim field notes They are transcribed using an adaptation of transcription conventions developed by Gail Jefferson (Atkinson and Heritage 1984). I use modified or outdated conventions because I do not want to convey an unwarranted sense of precision to my notations.

Single parentheses ( ) are used to indicate utterances or portions of utterances that were not reproduced verbatim. Some of these were inaudible or unclear, so the parentheses include my estimation of what was said. Segments of talk that passed by too quickly to be precisely recorded are presented within parentheses in summarized and condensed form. My attempt is to characterize the essence of the talk as I recalled it.

Double parentheses (( )) contain characterizations of features of talk like silences and audible inflections. Indicating silences in my field notes was problematic. I noted all silences I perceived, but short pauses within and between utterances were undoubtedly imperceptible under the circumstances. For a silence to be noted, its duration would have been *approximately* one second or more. When silences were extended, I attempted to *estimate* and note their length. Silences were approximately one to three seconds in duration when estimates of length are not noted.

Double slashes (//) indicate the *approximate* onset of simultaneous speech by the next speaker. Because these are field notes and not transcriptions of recorded talk, the precision of my notations is problematic. // marks the *general* location where I estimate that the succeeding line of speech intrudes upon the current line. Many minor instances of simultaneous speech that I could not note undoubtedly occurred.

Square brackets [ ] contain clarifications or additional information supplied by the author to help the reader understand the context of the recorded talk.

Ellipsis points (. . .) are used to indicate that I have omitted words, portions of utterances, or complete utterances for the sake of brevity, or because they could not be recorded.

2.   It was not uncommon, especially in Metropolitan Court, for DAs to ask doctors who might not appear to be, or sound like, native-born Americans (i.e., nonwhite, audibly accented speech) to state their place of birth, give their educational history, describe the institutions where they received their medical training, and indicate how long they had been in the United States and where and how long they had been in psychiatric practice.

3.   In California, the law requires the treating physician to make the psychiatric assessment in court. The attorneys in Metropolitan Court—with the judge's cooperation—"stipulate" that qualified staff members from the treating facility may testify in the absence of the treating physician. This is a pragmatic agreement that allows a single physician from a facility to appear in court to testify in several commitment cases involving the facility's patients.

Regular personnel typically honor the agreement to allow doctors other than the treating physician to testify. They do, however, routinely question the testifying doctor in such instances regarding his or her familiarity with the case at hand, seeking indications that the doctor's psychiatric assessment might somehow be flawed by not having worked with the actual patient. PDs regularly argue that the medicolegal assessments made by nontreating doctors may not adequately consider those factors beyond psychiatric diagnosis that must figure into assessments of danger or grave disability.

4.   Note that in the sequence the PD refrained from drawing this conclusion, but punctuated the series of questions with an extended silence (line 14) that invited listeners to reflect upon the implications of the preceding answers given by the doctor. Chapter 5 discusses in greater detail some of the implications of silences for the production of testimony.

5.   In those cases where the PD declined to call a witness, the judge typically expressed surprise or inquired, "Are you sure?" marking the occasion as a conscious omission rather than an oversight or an indication of some other

problem with the proceedings. His remarks made it clear that the patient had been given the opportunity to present his or her case in court.

6. These issues and other techniques DAs use to produce psychiatric symptoms will be discussed in detail in Chapter 5.

7. Another noteworthy aspect of legal proceedings like commitment hearings is the legal requirement that testimony and argument be produced so that it may be recorded. The production of a transcript of the proceedings marks hearings as legally sanctioned occasions.

Chapter 5

The Conversational Organization of
Competence and Incompetence

Involuntary commitment hearings are occasions when deviance designations and remedial responses are *publicly* assembled, made sensible,
challenged, and defended. Psychiatric experts, for example, invariably
testify that patients are seriously ill, supporting their diagnoses with
descriptions of disturbed, disruptive, or delusional thoughts and behaviors. In cases charging grave disability and, in some instances, danger to self, psychiatrists often support their commitment recommendations by arguing that patients' mental disturbances have rendered them
socially and interactionally incompetent. This incompetence—often
phrased as the inability to "negotiate the routine transactions of everyday life," or to "get along with other people," and similar vernacular
characterizations—is cited as grounds for hospitalization.

The prevailing interpretation of commitment laws emphasizes practical as well as medical reasons for hospitalization. Mental illness must
result in some type of consequential social impairment or disturbance
for hospitalization to be warranted. So, while psychiatric diagnoses are
typically accepted without challenge, the consequences of patients' mental illness are often made problematic. With this in mind, PDs and DAs
indicate that as they interrogate patients, they try to elicit firsthand
evidence of interactional competence and incompetence, respectively.
While expert testimony is crucial, the court looks to patients themselves
for witnessable indications of interactional capability and impairment,
scrutinizing both the substance of patients' testimony and the manner in
which that testimony is delivered. Talk is thought to index patients'
more general abilities to function in everyday circumstances.

This chapter analyzes the interactional production of some of the
putative documents of competence and incompetence that are said to
be characteristic or "symptomatic" of patients' conditions. Rather than

treating them as individuals' characteristics, however, it analyzes them as accomplishments achieved in cooperation with others. While competence and incompetence are commonsensically attributed only to the person whose commitment is under consideration, close examination of courtroom interaction suggests that the documents of competence and incompetence result from *collaboration* between the patients and other hearing participants. Thus, what are generally construed as signs of individual deviance or normalcy are joint productions (Holstein 1988a).

Interactional Competence and "Crazy Talk"

Most hearing participants agree that a sure sign of incompetence that often emerges in courtroom proceedings is "crazy talk." Talk considered delusional, disoriented, or bizarre is said to interfere with social functioning, as one Metropolitan Court judge noted: "If their [patients'] talk gets so crazy, so delusional that it makes no sense, it tells me that they won't be able to make it very far if I release them." A Southern Court judge concurred: "If they can't manage to make themselves sound reasonable when they know their freedom is on the line, what can we expect them to do when they're on their own?"

"Crazy talk" is identified in terms of both content and form. Talk that others claim is disorganized to the point of being unintelligible may be described using vernacular or pseudotechnical terms like *crazy, schizophrenic, incomprehensible,* and *word salad*. Claims or reports that violate "known-in-common" understandings of times, places, and identities are also considered crazy. For example, patients routinely claim that they are or that they have consorted with movie stars or other entertainment celebrities (e.g., John Wayne, Richard Pryor, Janis Joplin), world leaders and statesmen (e.g., John F. Kennedy, Ronald Reagan, Fidel Castro), religious figures (e.g., Jesus Christ, the Pope, Martin Luther King), fictional characters (e.g., James Bond, Rocky Balboa, Lois Lane) and other well-known personalities, both dead and alive. Some patients also claim to see, hear, or experience things that "normal" others allegedly cannot experience (e.g., speaking with dead persons or extraterrestrials, seeing visions, or hearing voices that others cannot perceive).

Such claims fall outside the bounds of categories supported by our culturally grounded systems of verification (Coulter 1973)—those things that we all have good reason to "know to be true or possible," and "know that everyone else knows to be true" as well. Consequently, they engender serious doubt, if not disbelief. Disputed perceptual accounts may be analyzed as "interpretive asymmetries" (Coulter 1975) or "reality disjunctures" (Pollner 1975, 1987). Rational actors in the world of everyday life assume that a singular reality exists "out there," which is internally consistent and which can be truly known by following procedures of rational inquiry (Pollner 1987). Pollner argues that this assumption is incorrigible; discrepancies are invariably resolved so as to preserve the integrity of the idealization. Consequently, when conflicting claims are made, account recipients interpret and reconcile them by using forms of "mundane reason" that preserve the assumption of an objective, commonly shared world. Reality disjunctures are explained by formulating at least one of the discrepant accounts as the product of an exceptional method of observation, experience, or reporting (Pollner 1975). Ascribing insanity (in its many vernacular as well as technical usages) is one method of reconciling implausible accounts, casting at least one of the claims as the product of defective or distortive psychological mechanisms. Hence, when bizarre talk emerges in commitment hearings, its hearers are likely to make sense of it by casting it as crazy, a product of mental illness.

While courtroom participants utilize vernacular interpretations of insanity or mental illness, the isomorphism between vernacular and technical usage is sufficient to satisfy the practical purposes at hand. Participants acknowledge that their understandings are often nontechnical (although they are highly informed by the unrelenting psychiatric discourse of the commitment hearing environment), but trust that their own interpretations accord sufficiently with actual psychiatric conditions that they freely engage in vernacular characterizations throughout the proceedings. And because perceivedly crazy talk is said to be so revealing and consequential, DAs and PDs attend closely to its production and orient their questioning to its appearance, even though establishing direct evidence of mental illness or sanity on the witness stand is not required by commitment laws.

Judges and other court personnel also infer competence and incompetence from the manner in which patients deliver their testimony. That is, they attend to the *form* of patients' courtroom conversation for what they believe are indicators of interactional abilities or dysfunctions. Judges' accounts for commitment decisions routinely cite conversational disfluencies as evidence that patients cannot interact normally and competently. As one judge noted, "I look at how they communicate. If they're all messed up, real jumpy, if they're not able to answer the questions or put things together in complete sentences." Another said, "I'm looking to see if they can carry on a smooth conversation without a lot of stammering and stuttering, gibberish, and the like."

Judges also say they scrutinize patients' responses to questioning, taking direct, prompt, and appropriate answers as indications of social and conversational skill. However, judges cite unwillingness or inability to answer questions, as well as hesitations, false starts, and restarts as signs that a patient has trouble conversing, hence, interacting with others. As judges indicate, lapses in "getting their act together" or "getting their story straightened out" are convincing documents of interactional problems. Judges thus infer incompetence, and possibly grave disability, from such conversational difficulties and failures.

Troubles in courtroom talk can be assigned a variety of plausible causes, for example, lack of knowledge, anxiety, momentary confusion, or even lying. But in commitment hearings, mental illness is clearly the most likely account to be offered. This is due, at least partly, to the interpretive predisposition embedded in the ongoing membership categorization of the "mental patient" or "mentally ill person." According to Sacks (1972), a person who has been categorized by means of a particular device is likely to be further interpreted according to the properties of that category, in the interest of both consistency and economy. Thus, when witnesses produce problematic talk, their status as "mental patients" (as well as the psychiatric discourse that characterizes commitment hearings) influences others to hear the troublesome talk as documents of mental disturbance and incompetence, rather than signs of some other sort of difficulty.

Recognizing that judges are concerned with conversational difficulties, and sharing the belief that displayed difficulties signify deeper problems, DAs and PDs formulate their questions so as to create conversational environments in which patients are most likely to reveal themselves in desired ways. PDs and DAs thus employ different questioning practices and procedures for soliciting patients' testimony, PDs looking for competence while DAs seek disturbance.

Organizing Interactional Competence

As they interrogate patients, PDs pursue a variety of objectives, including directly rebutting the previously offered psychiatric assessment. One aspect of their strategy is to encourage the patient to show that he or she is not as disabled, incapacitated, or disruptive as the doctor previously claimed. PDs try to elicit coherent, responsive testimony that demonstrates the sort of interactional competence that judges require for release to be a viable option. Conversely, PDs are reluctant to call witnesses who are actively delusional, who display florid symptoms, or who cannot deliver coherent, intelligible testimony. They argue that calling witnesses who are likely to behave in these fashions simply confirms the psychiatrists' accusations. Of course, not calling the patient to the witness stand was a virtual concession to hospitalization because court personnel all assumed that a patient who did not testify was incapable of doing so in a rational manner.

When time allowed, PDs generally tried to instruct their clients regarding how they should comport themselves on the witness stand and how they should answer questions. Especially in Metropolitan Court, they were likely to begin by telling their clients to "just relax and tell the judge what you want to say." But they also suggested that the witness try to answer questions as directly and concisely as possible: "Just answer the questions we're going to ask you and don't say anything else." This "coaching" could be quite extensive, as PDs would run through possible questions and answers the patient might need to consider.

PDs try to make their interrogations as simple and straightforward as possible, attempting to facilitate coherent responses from their clients. The following example is a segment of the direct examination of a patient who had been instructed before her hearing in a fairly standard fashion. The PD told her, "Just stick to the questions. I'll ask you some things, and you just give me the answers." The sequence typifies the PDs' desire to "keep it simple."

[5:1] [Metropolitan Court; J2, DA4, PD4, Dr9, Katie Maxwell]

1.	PD4:	If they let you go today, Katie, do you have a place to live?
2.	KM:	Uh huh my mother's (place)
3.	PD4:	Where is your mother's place?
4.	KM:	In Bellwood.
5.	PD4:	What's the address?
6.	KM:	One twenty Acton Street. I can come // and go as I please.
7.	PD4:	((breaking in)) That's fine Katie.
8.		Does your mother say you can live with her?
9.	KM:	Yeah it's OK with her.
10.	PD4:	Can you eat your meals there?
11.	KM:	Yeah there's no one there // always watching me.
12.	PD4:	((breaking in)) You can just answer yes or no. OK?
13.	KM:	OK.
14.	PD4:	Do you have clothes at your mother's house?
15.	KM:	Yes.
16.	PD4:	Can you dress yourself?
17.	KM:	Of course I can.
18.	PD4:	Do you get an (SSI) check in the mail?
19.	KM:	Yes.
20.	PD4:	Will you give it to your mother?
21.	KM:	Yes.
22.	PD4:	And will you let her give you your medication?
23.	KM:	Yeah, whenever I // need it.
24.	PD4:	((breaking in)) That's good Katie.

The PD's questions clearly focused on formal grave disability criteria, raising issues of residence, food, clothing, medication, financial support, and security. At the same time, the segment of talk reveals a set of conversational practices that promote the *forms* of talk the PD wanted her client to display. Note, for example, how the PD's questions were formulated to elicit brief, direct answers. All but one (line 5) were answerable in a single word. The PD established the adequacy of such answers both explicitly, by instructing the witness to simply answer "yes or no" (line 12), and tacitly, by accepting brief answers as complete and moving directly to the next question without hesitation. Speaker transition was immediate as the PD claimed her preallocated turn.

When Ms. Maxwell attempted to elaborate her answers, however, the PD broke into her talk. In three instances (lines 6, 11, and 23), Maxwell tried to embellish or qualify her minimal answer to the PD's question, and each time the embellishments met with intrusions of simultaneous speech. The content of each overlapping utterance indicated that the patient's answer was adequately completed (e.g., line 7: "That's fine Katie."). Just as significantly, the incursions into the patient's turns discouraged continuation. The PD thus managed the patient's talk to accomplish the appearance of concise, direct testimony. She organized her questions to constrain the patient's answers at the first possible turn completion point (see Sacks, Schegloff, and Jefferson 1974), trying to keep testimony directly responsive to the questions asked.

PDs vigilantly anticipated crazy talk. In extract [5:1], when Ms. Maxwell began to elaborate answers at lines 6, 11, and 23, the PD immediately broke in, competing for speakership perhaps as a precaution against Maxwell's production of inappropriate answers. On other occasions when talk that might have been heard as crazy or inappropriate began to emerge, PDs moved quickly to terminate it, as in the following instances.

[5:2]   [Metropolitan Court; J1, DA3, PD1, Dr13, Fred Smitz]

1.   PD1:   Where would you live?
2.   FS: I think I'd go to a new board and care home not populated by
3.   rapists // and Iranian agents.
4.   PD1:   ((breaking in)) Fine, Mister Smitz now would you take your
5.   medication?
6.   FS: I would if it didn't pass//through the hands of too many Russians.
7.   PD1:   ((breaking in)) Do you get an SSI check Mister Smitz?

[5:3]   [Metropolitan Court; J1, DA5, PD6, Dr21, Roger Madison]

1.   PD6:   Will you go to the Mental Health Center for your medicine?
2.   RM: I'll try unless unless // unless the voices get too loud.
3.   PD6:   ((breaking in)) And you'll take it like the doctor says?

In [5:2], the patient offered an apparently appropriate answer in line 2, but began to introduce referents that were hearable as delusions. The PD broke in, using the patient's name to refocus his attention, then moved immediately to a new question about medication. In line 6, the patient answered and again began a qualification that culminated in a hearably delusional reference. The PD simultaneously produced another new question. Similar practices appear in [5:3], where an extended answer met with simultaneous, hence constraining, speech. The effect of these intrusions was to override, if not obliterate, the seemingly inappropriate talk that was beginning to emerge. Development of topics offered in crazy utterances was aggressively constrained as the PDs attempted to manage the content of what was being said.

PDs sometimes responded to inappropriate talk by "not responding," as in the following extract.

[5:4]   [Metropolitan Court; J1, DA2, PD2, Dr11, Irene Perez]

1.	PD2:	Do you want to leave the hospital?
2.	IP:	Yes, I do. Yeah.
3.	PD2:	If you do will you live with your parents?
4.	IP:	Yes.
5.	PD2:	Will they let you stay with them?
6.	IP:	Yes.
7.	PD2:	Will you eat (your meals) at home?
8.	IP:	Yes, except when I go out to dinner with my boyfriend
9.		Gabriel, he's the Christ.
10.	PD2:	Are all your clothes at home?
11.	IP:	Yes.
12.	PD2:	Do you think you'll be happy living at home?
13.	IP:	I think so.
14.	PD2:	What will you do for money?
15.	IP:	There's no such thing as money.
16.	PD2:	Will you take your medicine like you're supposed to?

Twice in this exchange (lines 8–9 and 15), Ms. Perez answered questions in ways that might be heard as delusional. While the PD failed to break in on either occasion (as the PDs did in the three examples above), he *immediately* continued his questioning, moving away from the inappropriate testimony by asking questions that did not deal with the content of the prior utterances (lines 10 and 16). The PD declined to focus on the provocative responses, thus minimizing the impact of the inappropriate answers by immediately posing new questions.[1]

Ignoring inappropriate talk, then, is a way of managing seemingly damaging talk. PDs did not acknowledge that they had explicit strategies for dealing with crazy talk in this fashion. Rather, they indicated that they sometimes "get caught off guard" by their clients' testimony and simply have to forge ahead with their questioning. As one PD said, "You never know when they'll say something crazy, so you just have to go ahead and make the best of it, hope they don't blow it altogether."

Thus, while the *content* of the testimony in cases like [5:4] may undermine the PD's argument against commitment, the form of the exchange between attorney and client is impeccable. Questions generate responses. Responses are accepted as answers and the interrogation proceeds smoothly. Transition from one speaker to another is achieved in an orderly fashion with minimal overlap between speakers and without gap between adjacent turns—characteristics of competent everyday conversation (Sacks et al. 1974). The patient might still appear conversationally competent, even though the content of his or her speech was hearably delusional. PDs are thus able to manage the form, if not the content of testimony, allowing for the possible hearing of coherence in talk that might otherwise seem incompetent.

Organizing Incompetence

When DAs cross-examine patients, they try to deflate the patients' rebuttals of prior psychiatric assessments and undermine their claims of fitness for release. To this end, DAs concentrate on the practical details of how patients will secure food, clothing, and shelter, but they also attempt to elicit factual discrepancies and hearably unreasonable claims that might expose vulnerabilities in patients' cases. In addition, they try to elicit crazy talk that they feel proves irrefutably that the patient cannot function adequately in social situations. In their own fashion, DAs are as conscientious as PDs in managing cross-examination speech exchanges to achieve their objectives, to have patients display behaviors that might be construed as interactional incompetence. If a patient exhibits behavior that could be seen as symptomatic, DAs can subsequently argue that no deinstitutionalized setting could provide adequate care and security for a person so deranged and hence so disabled.[2] DAs, then, attempt to produce a conversational environment conducive to testimony that reveals, either in content or form, that patients are incapable of normal interactions.

Producing Contradictions

One common interrogation strategy is to promote contrasts and contradictions between patients' testimony and the psychiatric assessments offered by the doctors who examined them. As noted in Chapter 4, DAs establish psychiatrists as qualified experts through elaborate sequences of questions regarding their credentials and experience. They are the first witnesses called and provide elaborate testimony and medical reasoning to document their diagnoses and recommendations. PDs, in concert with their clients, try to counter these assessments through testimony and direct behavioral evidence. When DAs cross-examine patients, however, they often ask them to provide their own psychiatric assessments, looking for responses that can then be juxtaposed with the assessment previously offered by the psychiatrists, as in the following exchanges.

[5:5] [Metropolitan Court; J1, DA3, PD1, Dr5, Mel Collins]

1. DA3: Do you have any mental problems?
2. MC: No I'm OK.
3. DA3: Doctor Lee's examined you and she seems to think you aren't OK.
4.   Why do you think she says you're mentally ill?
5. MC: She's lying. She's probably trying to get me.
6.   How does she know anyway?

[5:6] [Metropolitan Court; J2, DA5, PD6, Dr20, Ruth Shirley]

1. DA5: The doctor says you're pretty sick. Do you agree?
2. RS: I got my problems but I'm not crazy.
3. DA5: Well that's not what he says. Why do you think you have so many
4.   problems?
5. RS: I don't have so many problems. Other people just have a problem
6.   with me. It's their problem.
7. DA5: So you're not schizophrenic?
8. RS: Not hardly.
9. DA5: And you're not delusional?
10. RS: What I know is real.
11. DA5: And you haven't heard voices talking to you?
12. RS: I've heard voices, but they're real.

The question in line 1 of [5:5] presents a dilemma for the patient. To answer affirmatively would imply agreement with arguments for hospitalization, while denial places the witness at odds with prior expert testimony. The DA refers to that testimony in line 3, discrediting the denial of mental illness. He produces a visible discrepancy between Mr. Collins's perspective and that of the psychiatric authority, a reality disjuncture that begs resolution. The DA offers Mr. Collins an opportunity to resolve the disjuncture in line 4, and Mr. Collins responds by calling Dr. Lee a liar. The response does deal with the disjuncture by trying to invalidate the doctor's testimony, but whatever it might indicate about the patient's mental status, it is also an insult to a witness whose legitimacy has been certified by the court.

Extract [5:6] is a similar sequence in which the patient's judgment is at odds with the expert witness's. While such testimony might be interpreted as a countervailing claim that legitimately attempts to refute the doctor's assessment, in commitment hearings it is likely to have the opposite effect. In [5:6], the DA reports the expert's opinion, then solicits Ms. Shirley's view on the matter (line 1). Her response in line 2 directly contradicts the doctor's. The subsequent series of questions refers to various aspects of the doctor's diagnosis, and Ms. Shirley's responses all conflict with the doctor's claims. Once again, a series of contradictions invites explanation.

Reality disjunctures like these may be resolved by invoking the membership categories of contending parties to warrant the acceptance of one version over the other. The court has invested considerable time and procedure in establishing the credibility of the psychiatrist, so his or her membership in the *expert* category may weight the resolution in the direction of his or her claim. At the same time, patients have explicitly been assigned to the *mentally ill* category. Any claim by a member of this category is implicitly suspect. Moreover, there is a compelling account for the patient's discrepant testimony available in the *mental illness* category itself. Coulter (1975) suggests that hearers may assign fault for the production of "interpretive asymmetries" by aligning an appropriate fault category with a membership category.

In extracts [5:5] and [5:6], the patients' "mentally ill" or "schizophrenic" status makes the *delusional* fault category readily available as a framework for understanding the disagreement with the psychiatrist. In commitment hearings, the use of this category may be more appropriate or compelling than explaining the discrepant reports as the doctors' diagnostic errors, or simple mistakes or lies on the part of the patients. In the developing context, judges are unlikely to resolve the reality disjuncture in favor of patients' claims, which challenge the established courtroom order and are readily discountable as *delusions*. Rather, judges may use psychiatric diagnoses to warrant interpretive resolutions that further confirm patients' mental illness. Consequently, patient testimony that contradicts expert opinion is not treated as a countervailing report, but instead is seen as a symptom itself.

Soliciting "Crazy Talk"

DAs have a second objective when asking patients to comment on their own symptoms, delusions, or problematic conduct. Raising the subject of delusions, hallucinations, or other bizarre instances may prompt patients to focus on the subject, sometimes getting them to display the very behaviors that the DA asked about. In the following examples, DAs simply asked patients to speak about delusions that had been noted either in psychiatric testimony or in the patients' medical records.

[5:7]   [Midland Court; J1, DA1, PD2, Dr2, Doris Waleski]

1.   DA1:   The doctor says that you have delusions, that you've spoken to
2.   the Pope. Have you?
3.   DW: We've talked. I go to the church and we talk. People don't
4.   believe me but he's a very nice man.

[5:8]   [Metropolitan Court; J1, DA5, PD4, Dr4, Jason Andro]

1.   DA5:   The doctor says you've been calling yourself Hercules. Why?
2.   JA: Look at me. I look like Hercules don't I? I am the one . . .
3.   DA5:   Haven't you said that your brother is Jesus Christ?
4.   JA: Yes I think so. Ever since he was born I could see he was
5.   Christ. I guess I saw this when I was about eighteen. About
6.   four years ago.
7.   DA5:   Are you sure?
8.   JA: As sure as I can be.
9.   DA5:   But didn't you also say that your mother was the devil?
10. JA: Yes. I've seen it in her eyes.

Sometimes questions like these prompted denials. Such responses, however, place the witness in direct conflict with expert testimony and invite the sort of interpretive vulnerabilities discussed in the preceding section. Answers like those in [5:7] and [5:8], however, are even more likely to be cited in support of arguments to commit. In each case, the patient responded to inquiries about putatively delusional behavior with answers that were themselves hearably crazy. By making mental illness topical, the DAs often elicited spates of crazy talk that demonstrated firsthand the very delusions that were being discussed.

"Letting Them Hang Themselves"

DAs typically feel that patients will "reveal" symptoms of mental disorder and interactional dysfunction if they are simply allowed to speak without constraint. To promote this, DAs routinely engage in a practice they refer to as "letting them hang themselves." According to one DA, this consists of "getting them up there [on the witness stand] and just letting them talk. You don't really have to do anything." DAs indicate that if allowed to talk freely, patients will almost invariably "hang themselves," "do themselves in," or "make the case against themselves." "You let them talk and they hospitalize themselves," noted one DA. DAs thus suggest that patients inevitably and voluntarily display the kinds of talk that judges, DAs, and psychiatrists cite as documents of mental disorder: hearably delusional, disorganized, incoherent, fragmented, or discontinuous utterances.

Patients do talk more during cross-examinations than under direct examination, and crazy talk is more common. These differences can be at least partly explained by reference to the structure of the interactional sequences that produce patients' testimony. As noted above, PDs question patients in ways that promote brief answers and discourage elaborations. In contrast, while DAs claim that they merely "let them [patients] talk," their interrogation encourages more expansive testimony. "Letting them hang themselves" is a complex of conversation practices that invites patients to produce extended utterances containing talk that may be interpreted as crazy.

In [5:9] below, for example, the DA introduced a line of questioning that he acknowledged in a later interview to be an instance of "letting her talk until she got herself committed." After initiating fourteen prior question-answer pairs (one immediately following the other) regarding the patient's intended residence and who she planned to live with, the DA changed tactics:

[5:9]   [Metropolitan Court; J1, DA2, PD2, Dr12, Lisa Sellers]

1.	DA2:	How do you like summer out here, Lisa?
2.	LS:	It's OK.
3.	DA2:	How long have you lived here?
4.	LS:	Since I moved from Houston.
5.		((silence))³
6.	LS:	About three years ago.
7.	DA2:	Tell me about why you came here.
8.	LS:	I just came.
9.		((silence))
10.	LS:	You know, I wanted to see the stars, Hollywood.
11.		((silence))
12.	DA2:	Uh huh.
13.	LS:	I didn't have no money.
14.		((silence))
15.	LS:	I'd like to get a good place to live.
16.		((silence five seconds))
17.	DA2:	Go on. ((spoken simultaneously with onset of next utterance))
18.	LS:	There was some nice things I brought.
19.		((silence))
20.	DA2:	Uh huh.

21.   LS: Brought them from the rocketship.
22.   DA2:   Oh really?
23.   LS: They was just some things I had.
24.   DA2:   From the rocketship?
25.   LS: Right.
26.   DA2:   Were you on it?
27.   LS: Yeah.
28.   DA2:   Tell me about this rocketship, Lisa.

The sequence culminates in Ms. Sellers's hearably delusional references to a rocketship, from the DA's point of view, a successful instance of "letting them hang themselves." Throughout the exchange, the DA encouraged Ms. Sellers to take extended and unfocused turns at talk by removing many of the constraints supplied by the PD who had previously questioned her. First, he altered the normal or expected sequence of question-answer adjacency pairs. In the fourteen exchanges immediately prior to this extract, and continuing in lines 1 through 4, the DA asked a question, then followed Ms. Sellers's answers with additional questions, allowing no notable gaps between answers and next questions. A silence, however, followed line 4, where a question from the DA may have been expected. The gap in talk was eventually terminated (line 6) by Ms. Sellers's elaboration of her prior utterance.

In line 7, the DA solicited further talk, but not in the form of a question. Instead, he made a very general request for more information, but the adequacy of a response to this form of solicit was more indeterminate than to a directly asked question. The DA's discretion is deeply implicated here in what may come to be seen as adequately fulfilling the request, the completeness of a response depending, in part, on how he acknowledges it. The DA did not respond at the first possible speaker transition point after Ms. Sellers's next utterance (lines 8 and 9), declining possible speakership or filling turnspaces with minimal acknowledgments or solicits through line 20. Ms. Sellers's mention of a rocketship finally elicited an indication of apparent interest ("Oh really?") from the DA at line 22, and a subsequent set of questions pursuing the subject.[4]

This type of response marks a significant noticing that might accomplish several things. First, it can focus attention on the prior utterance so as to invite further talk on the subject. Such noticings may also call attention to a "faulted" quality of an utterance, suggesting the need for repair. In extract [5:9], when the DA responded to Ms. Sellers's statement about the rocketship, his use of "Oh really?" (line 22) could be heard as an expression of surprise or disbelief, a call for elaboration that invited Ms. Sellers to dispel implied doubts by altering, repairing, retracting, or reframing the problematic utterance. Her indifference to the opportunity to retract or explain the claim may be interpreted as further evidence that she was incapable of recognizing and correcting conversational "gaffes" that any competent interactant would probably not make, and certainly would repair, if given the opportunity.[5]

Clearly, this testimony, like other extended multiunit turns at talk, is an interactional achievement (Schegloff 1982, 1987). The DA requested testimony from the patient, but repeatedly withheld acknowledgment of the testimony's adequacy, promoting more unfocused talk in the process. He further encouraged Ms. Sellers to speak, using "Uh huh" to indicate an understanding that an extended unit of talk was in progress and was not yet complete (Schegloff 1982), and by declining possible turns at talk altogether. He resumed an active role in the dialogue only after hearably crazy talk emerged, at which point he attempted to focus the discussion on the crazy topic and encourage Ms. Sellers to elaborate. For her part, Ms. Sellers sustained the ongoing conversation by terminating silences that had begun to emerge at failed speaker transition points. She repeatedly elaborated responses, and eventually produced the crazy talk that was cited as evidence of her interactional incompetence. But, in a sense, it was her cooperation with the DA in extending the conversation—her conversational *competence*—that allowed for the emergence of that very talk.

Focusing "Crazy Talk"

DAs' role in the production of crazy talk is evident in the way they manage conversational focus. As long as patients' testimony is perceivedly normal, DAs' participation is typically limited to soliciting information and facilitating continued talk, often with minimal, neutral acknowledgments that a response had been given and accepted. But as we see in extract [5:9], crazy talk was frequently highlighted and promoted by change-of-state tokens and newsmarks (Heritage 1984) that focused attention on selected segments of talk. This can also be seen in the following extracts.

[5:10]   [Metropolitan Court; J1, DA1, PD3, Dr4, Ralph Lange]

1.   1RL: I can hear all of your thoughts on my mind radio.
2.   DA1:   Oh, yeah?
3.   RL: Everything. I can tune you in and out.

[5:11]   [Metropolitan Court; J1, DA3, PD3, Dr10, Carmen Hidalgo]

1.   CH: I'm a doctor and a nurse. I delivered a thousand babies myself.
2.   DA3:   Oh, you did?
3.   CH: Yes and that was only last year.

Each of these extracts followed sequences of questions, responses, requests to continue, and further responses (similar to extract [5:9]). The DAs began to focus the conversation only after hearably crazy utterances emerged. These crazy utterances are a type of incipient news announcement—that is, currently incomplete reports on activities that are speaker related and recipient relevant (Button and Casey 1985). Such announcements project particular sequential relevancies for the next turn at talk. Next turns may topicalize the news, providing the occasion to elaborate upon the original announcement. Crazy talk— announcements of incomprehensible activity, for example—was invariably highlighted and encouraged by the use of conversational markers that drew attention to the crazy utterance, signaled its newsworthiness, and invited further talk by the patient.

"Oh," as it was used in the cases above, proposes that its speaker has undergone a change in his or her current state of knowledge, awareness, or orientation. It marks a significant noticing, that, when tied to newsmarks ("Oh, yeah?" "Oh, you did?"), invites further informing and/or explanation (Heritage 1984). Indeed, these noticings provide both opportunity and warrant to repair or clarify the utterance that has been highlighted, if not questioned. A failure to clarify, "normalize," or account for the hearably crazy utterance is understandable as a further lapse in competence, and may be cited as confirmatory evidence of interactional dysfunction. When a patient is given the opportunity, for example, to retract, rephrase, or interpret a claim that he is Jesus Christ or President John F. Kennedy, and this sort of response is not forthcoming, he provides two bases for subsequent charges of incompetence. First, he has made an implausible or incomprehensible claim, and, second, he has failed to capitalize on the structured opportunity to neutralize or undo the arguably damaging statement.

DAs routinely respond to problematic utterances in ways that make the talk salient and encourage its continuation. Crazy talk, then, is not attributable to the patient alone. It is a conversational accomplishment that owes its emergence, at least in part, to the *interactional* work of *both* its participants. The "seen but unnoticed" character of its joint production, however, leaves the craziness of the discourse attributable only to the patient, whom the court holds responsible as its sole author.

Producing Disjointed Talk

In addition to encouraging patients to elaborate their turns at talk, DAs also contribute to a speech environment that invites repeated shifts in the focus of the testimony. This is doubly consequential for patients who are trying to demonstrate their interactional competence. First, continually shifting lines of talk increases the likelihood of saying something crazy. Second, repeated shifts can provide for an extended turn or series of turns that sounds discontinuous or fragmented—that is, *incoherent* conversation. To the extent that such unfocused talk is attributed to the patient, he or she may be perceived as conversationally disfluent or incompetent.

Extract [5:12] below is a segment of cross-examination that the judge claimed revealed the patient's "mental incompetence." In his account for hospitalizing Henry Johnson on the grounds of grave disability, the judge noted that Mr. Johnson's testimony was "confused and jumbled." As the judge put it, "He didn't know what to say. He was stopping and starting, jumping from one thing to another. You can see that he can't focus on one thing at a time." A portion of Mr. Johnson's testimony is extracted.

[5:12]   [Metropolitan Court; J1, DA4, PD1, Dr7, Henry Johnson]

1.	DA4:	How you been feeling lately?
2.	HJ:	OK.
3.		((silence))
4.	HJ:	I been feeling pretty good.
5.		((silence))
6.	DA4:	Uh huh.
7.		((silence))
8.	HJ:	Pretty good, ummm all right.
9.		((silence))
10.	HJ:	Got a job with (several words inaudible).
11.		((silence))
12.	HJ:	Pays OK, not bad.
13.		((silence four seconds))
14.	HJ:	My car got hit, an accident, really messed it up.
15.		((silence))
16.	HJ:	Got to get it on the street.
17.		((silence five seconds))
18.	HJ:	They gonna let us go to the truck out front?
19.	DA4:	When you're all done here they might.

Talk is discontinuous and multifocused in this example, a speech environment characterized by failed speaker transition and recurrent silence. In court, the talk was heard as an individual's production, and was interpreted as symptomatic or probative of the patient's interactional incompetence. But it is possible to consider this halting, disjointed movement from one line of talk to another as a *collaborative* phenomenon, framing discontinuous utterances as proffered solutions to the problems witnesses confront as they attempt to produce responsive testimony in a nonresponsive environment.

There is ample evidence that regular speaker transition, continuous conversation, and sustained topicality are interactional achievements rather than individual responsibilities (Sacks et al. 1974; Maynard 1980). One might argue that many cross-examination silences result from a DA's refusal to assume a turn or, at minimum, acknowledge hearably complete utterances by the patient, as in [5:12]. When Mr. Johnson offered topic-developmental utterances, the DA might have produced further questions, invitations, solicits, or continuers to sustain the line of talk. Even minimal utterances and solicits demonstrate recipient attention and invite further related talk (Maynard 1980). In the absence of these (as in lines 7–18), however, the line of talk may falter and silences may occur. Such silences may be heard as conversational difficulties, difficulties that implicate the prior speaker, who may attempt remedial action. One victim of a deteriorating line of talk is its topical continuity.

Topic changes (that is, utterances that utilize new referents and implicate and occasion new lines of talk unrelated to talk in prior turns) and topic shifts (lesser changes in the ongoing line of talk) are common solutions to problems of producing continuous talk (Maynard 1980). For example, utterances that fail to generate either speaker transition or solicits to continue may evoke silence. We can analyze the repeated silences in extracts [5:9] and [5:12] in these terms. Maynard (1980) suggests that participants encountering silences often try to restore continuous talk, first by pursuing the ongoing line of talk and then, if this fails, by changing the line of talk. In [5:12], Mr. Johnson discussed how he was feeling in three utterances (lines 2, 4, and 8). Continuation was explicitly encouraged only once (line 6). At line 10, Mr. Johnson shifted the line of talk, not abandoning the discussion of how he felt, but elaborating his reasons for his feelings. This line received no acknowledgment, but he continued the elaboration in a second utterance (line 12). When the DA was again nonresponsive, Mr. Johnson offered a new topic-developmental utterance, bringing up his recent automobile accident (line 14). This line and a subsequent elaboration (line 16) generated no response, and the testimony deteriorated into an extended silence. The patient ended the silence with another topical offering in the form of a question, explicitly inviting speaker transition (line 18). Extract [5:9] is similar, with the patient shifting the line of talk in response to failed speakership transfer and/or the DA's unwillingness to respond.

If we recognize an interactional basis for topical continuity, we cannot hold individual speakers solely responsible for maintaining a conversation's focus. As Maynard (1980) argues, topicality is constituted through joint conversational practices; it is more than a matter of content. Shifting the line of talk provides a procedural solution to problematic, nonresponsive speech environments. Changing the direction of the conversation, then, appears to be a pervasive and competent practice in environments characterized by repeated recipient silences. We encounter it frequently in patients' testimony, as they confront nonresponsive conversational partners—that is, DAs engaged in the practice of "letting them hang themselves." Analytically, we can appreciate this talk—talk that the court considers to be symptomatic of individuals' mental problems—as an interactional project.

Incompetence, Normalcy, and Conversational Practice

Commitment hearing participants cite patients' talk as evidence of their dysfunctions or normalcy in arguments both for and against commitment. Whereas these interactional documents are not the sole criteria for determining grave disability, they nonetheless compete with, and/or augment, other factors to which commitment decisions orient. And while attorneys acknowledge that they overtly manage witnesses' testimony, the commonsense evaluative procedures underpinning commitment hearings largely ignore the collaborative character of this testimony. Court personnel, for example, suggest that patients "respond better" to PDs than to DAs because PDs are known advocates who are more familiar and less threatening. We have seen, however, that the apparent coherence of direct examination testimony depends at least partially on the examination procedures themselves. Many of the PDs' questions are formulated to be answered in one word. Silences are not allowed to develop as PDs immediately claim their turn at talk at the earliest possible speaker transition point. Not only does this keep the conversation going, but it establishes the adequacy of patients' prior utterances as answers to prior questions (cf. West 1984).

The immediacy with which turns are claimed for next questions often results in PDs' talk overlapping patients' testimony. Such intrusions seal off the line of talk by reclaiming speakership for the PDs, and may be used to constrain crazy talk. Prompt speakership transfer also maintains a sense of continuity in patients' talk, minimizing silences and constraining shifts in the line of talk. PDs blend new topical offerings or crazy utterances into the ongoing exchange by reclaiming speakership as soon as possible and refocusing talk on less problematic topics, doing as little as possible to draw attention to the offending talk.

In contrast, DAs frequently engage patients in talk that is hearably disjointed and disorganized. DAs argue that their interrogation strategy merely provides patients with the opportunity to speak for themselves—to either "hospitalize themselves" or to "make their own case" for release. But in the course of eliciting this testimony, DAs ask relatively general questions, refuse numerous opportunities to claim turns, and respond minimally so as to invite continuation by the witness. Patients' talk is seldom overlapped. New topics are repeatedly offered, crazy talk is marked off for special attention, and these noteworthy lines of talk are encouraged. Some of patients' hearably incompetent or incoherent speech, then, is not merely of their own individual doing. Their testimony—their very talk—is produced *in concert* with their questioners.

In light of these observations, we might reconsider commonsense notions about the sources of interactional competence or incompetence. Both continuous and disjointed conversation, as well as topical speech, are plainly collaborative in many instances. When testimony is conceived to be as much an attorney's project as a witness's product, some segments of talk that are cited as incoherent or incompetent may be seen to display patients' responsive interactional activity, demonstrating their conversational proficiency. Similarly, the perceived competence of patients' direct-examination testimony might be attributed partly to the PDs who collaborated in its production.

Establishing competence and incompetence involves elaborate reality-creating and -sustaining practices. Indeed, it is evident that appearances of deviance and normalcy more generally are interactional products. Much as Lynch (1983) found "normal" appearances in mundane, everyday circumstances to be highly dependent upon collegial management of persons' public behaviors and impressions, data from involuntary commitment hearings demonstrate how seemingly "nonsymptomatic" conversation can be accomplished by the coordinated practices of partners in conversation. The methods through which PDs maneuvered their clients' talk are conversational examples of more general practices that are used to manage troublemakers and sustain a sense of normalcy about them in the course of everyday activity. Conversely, DAs' cross-examination procedures deeply implicate them in the production of perceivedly incompetent talk. The commonsense location of deviance or normalcy inside individuals thus glosses the interactional activity and conversational practice that make these phenomena visible.

* * * * *

Appearances of interactional competence and incompetence are clearly important to involuntary commitment proceedings, but alone they provide insufficient grounds for commitment decisions. Chapter 6 focuses on an alternative configuration of concerns relating to patients' troubles and the social circumstances they confront outside the hospital.

Notes

1. On some occasions when PDs believed that hospitalization was actually the best alternative for a client, they might be less attentive to constraining their clients' testimony. For example, in some cases where crazy talk began to emerge, PDs made little effort to contain or redirect inappropriate lines of talk. Indeed, the immediacy with which questions followed possibly complete answers in [5:2], [5:3], and [5:4] was sometimes replaced with hesitance in assuming the next turn, which might serve to invite even further crazy talk.

2. In fact, if a patient testified during direct examination in a hearably delusional, disorganized, or incoherent fashion, DAs often waived cross-examination, feeling that they did not need to demonstrate further need for hospitalization.

3. Indicating silences in my field notes was problematic. I noted all silences I perceived, but short pauses within and between utterances were undoubtedly imperceptible under the circumstances. For a silence to be noted, its duration would have been *approximately* one second or more. When silences were extended, I attempted to *estimate* and note their length. Silences were approximately one to three seconds in duration when estimates of length are not noted.

4. Note how the DA continued to exploit the topic of the rocketship with another general prompt (line 28: "Tell me about this rocketship, Lisa.") rather than a simple question, again promoting an open-ended discussion of the topic.

5. Extracts [5:10] and [5:11] display similar practices in responding to "noteworthy" testimony. In these instances, note the ways that expressions of newsworthiness focus the conversation.

Chapter 6

Troubles, Tenability, and the Placement of Insanity

While it is a legally necessary consideration in commitment decisions, mental illness is not sufficient grounds for involuntary hospitalization, either statutorily or as a matter of everyday practice. Because court personnel are convinced that all persons whose commitment is under consideration are mentally disturbed, they do not distinguish those who should be hospitalized from those who may be released on the basis of psychiatric condition. Instead, a constellation of concerns about material and social circumstances is deeply implicated in the interpretive practices that determine who shall be committed.

In his analysis of the "insanity of place," Goffman (1969) conceptualized symptoms of mental illness interactionally, framing them as products of circumstances in which one person is unable or unwilling to abide the local place others accord him or her. Conflicts over claims of place, if irreconcilable and incorrigible, profoundly disrupt the local social system, causing what Goffman calls "organizational havoc." Diagnoses or labels of mental illness provide definitional resolutions to such problems, while mental hospitalization offers practical solutions to the troubles. Involuntary commitment can be viewed as a remedy for havoc; it extrudes the mentally ill from the local social order because other community members are neither willing to honor the definitions, relational claims, rights, and responsibilities they assert, nor bear the burdens or risk the hazards they present.

Court personnel keenly appreciate the havoc associated with mental illness. Given their assumptions about patients' mental status, and the concern for doing something about the troubles at hand, commitment decision-making typically becomes a practical task of placing the "insane" in some social and/or physical environment that can contain or accommodate mental symptoms. The potential for havoc is weighed against the perceived capacity of a social setting to contain such havoc.

113

Community placement may be possible if adequate circumstances are available, but commitment is likely if the psychiatric ward proves the only viable place to accommodate the person in question. Commitment hearings, then, orient to the alternative ways of dealing with psychiatrically troubled and troublesome persons; the practical issue is the "placement of insanity" (Holstein 1984).

Tenability and Troubles

Research on mental hospitalization has increasingly converged on the notion that most mental patients are admitted to psychiatric hospitals because their situations in the community have become untenable (Gove 1970; Scott 1974). As Goffman suggests, hospitalization is a practical remedy for some kinds of social turmoil. Studies of the emergency apprehension and hospitalization of the mentally ill by police (Bittner 1967) and psychiatric emergency teams (Emerson 1989) note the extent to which decision-making focuses on the community context in which troubles are encountered. The orientation to social context and to the tenability of community circumstances also dominates commitment proceedings (Holstein 1984). While psychiatric concerns never fully recede, commitment decisions rest on other grounds, most importantly, factors relating to the viability of the situation in which a patient might be placed, and his or her ability to function in that situation.

Commonsense assumptions about how situational factors ameliorate or worsen psychiatric distress provide the basis for courtroom arguments regarding the tenability of patients' community living situations. Grave disability (as well as some charges of dangerousness) is thus established only within the context of the patient's envisioned life circumstances. Hearings orient to whether or not the patient's mental disturbance and conduct is, or could be made, manageable in a particular living arrangement. Arguments by attorneys and judges suggest that release is plausible if an arrangement can be established that can contain, absorb, or tolerate the mentally ill person's anticipated erratic, troublesome, havoc-wreaking behavior—a tenable situation for a person of this sort. As a Northern Court judge suggested:

[6:1]   [Northern Court; J1]

> A lot of persons are hospitalized because their home situations can't cope. There is nothing else to do with them. There is no alternative. It's not exactly their mental illness and it's not their dangerousness. It's their inability to care for themselves; the inability to hook onto someone else, or

some place that will look out for them—someplace or someone to keep things on an even keel.

Note how the explanation focuses almost entirely on situational contingencies and practical issue of living in the community. Psychiatric disturbance remains important, but is relegated to the background.

The viability of a patient's proposed living situation is thus a central issue in nearly all commitment cases. In evaluating the tenability of a patient's proposed living arrangement, commitment hearings commonly consider the following features of the situation and the patient's life in it:

1. The mentally ill person's ability to provide for, gain access to, and properly utilize life's basic necessities. Food, clothing, shelter, and medical care are major, but not exclusive concerns. Arguments consider whether the person has access to the material and personal resources necessary to maintain a viable life in the community. Dependable income is a central consideration.
2. The willing presence of someone in the person's vicinity who will serve competently as "caretaker," look after the well-being of the released patient, and intervene if the person begins to act in a threatening or dangerous manner.
3. The acceptance of remedial treatment as a routine element of released patients' community lives. Patients must be willing to cooperate in containing the debilitating or dangerous manifestations of their mental illness and show how their living arrangements will explicitly accommodate treatment.

These features of community life are intricately intertwined so that one can usually be established only in conjunction with the others. In the conspicuous absence of any one of these, the tenability of one's living situation becomes problematic, and arguments for release encounter resistance. The following sections discuss how participants in commitment proceedings describe, establish, and assess the features of living situations to which commitment hearings orient.

Managing Basic Necessities

The ability to provide basic necessities is a prime consideration in all commitment decisions relating to grave disability. Establishing a patient's inability to obtain necessities, however, is not a completely straightforward matter; to determine that a person is clearly not feeding, dressing, or grooming him- or herself demands that variations in personal style, preference, and taste be taken into account. Said one Metropolitan Court judge, "Every person has his own way of life. Many of these people don't care if they live on the street."

However, judgments of the material adequacy of one's life-style are not completely relative. Participants in commitment hearings use testimony regarding patients' behavior in the time immediately preceding their confinement and the time immediately preceding their hearing—which was spent on a hospital ward—to establish patients' ability to carry out everyday activities and manage a standard set of "necessities."[1] They generate answers to the following questions (and other related questions as well) to provide grounds for their arguments:

- Does the person eat regularly?
- Can he or she shop for and prepare food?
- Does the person dress him- or herself?
- Does the person have a place to stay?
- Is the person sleeping enough at night?

Recall, for example, an exchange originally presented in Chapter 3 (extract [3:1]) involving charges of grave disability. The DA initially asked the psychiatrist if he had examined the patient, Howard Kimel. After establishing that Mr. Kimel was mentally ill, the DA asked the psychiatrist if he thought Mr. Kimel as gravely disabled.

[6:2]   [Metropolitan Court; J1, DA2, PD5, Dr8, Howard Kimel]

DA2:   Now, in your opinion, would you say that Mr. Kimel is gravely disabled as a result of this mental disorder?

Dr8:   Yes, I'd have to say so. He's unable to provide adequate nutrition. He doesn't take care of himself, has nowhere to stay. He does bizarre things, disruptive things for no apparent reason. . . . He wanders from place to place, no home, no family, no permanent address. . . . He has no income, no job. He's mentally ill, and he can't provide for himself in his present condition. It's a clear case of gravely disabled. If he doesn't receive further treatment, he will certainly deteriorate, get even worse.

DA2:   So, you believe that Mr. Kimel meets the standards of LPS and should remain in the hospital.

Dr8:   That's my opinion.

Note that selected aspects of LPS were addressed, but not in a literal or technical fashion. Rather, a practical correspondence was indicated between general descriptions of Mr. Kimel's circumstances and elements of commitment legislation. The law itself was left unspecified, allowing it to be loosely attached to the case at hand, inferentially suggesting that the features of Mr. Kimel's life depicted by the psychiatrist were indeed relevant to the application of the law. LPS was thus invoked and specified in an ad hoc fashion; the law was elaborated through implicit suggestions of its violation. Such ad hoc practices are characteristic of the way that the meaning of rules and laws is continually developed as rule users encounter actual cases and find that they must display the rationality of their actions, choices, and decisions (Garfinkel 1967; Zimmerman and Wieder 1970). The psychiatrist formulated the practical meaning of LPS and grave disability as he described the case at hand. His account simultaneously suggested that a combination of factors rendered Mr. Kimel's living situation untenable for a severely disturbed person, linking the circumstances of untenability to the principles of the law.

Hearing participants display special interest in where the patient will live and how the patient will support him- or herself, including the most mundane features of how one gets and spends money. Judges are generally skeptical about a patient's ability to negotiating the routine transactions of everyday life—both social and financial. They also question patients' ability to sustain and utilize a source of income, even if the source can be established as stable and secure. This attitude critically influences judicial arguments regarding those who contend they will support themselves through employment.

Mentally ill persons are assumed to behave erratically, and are at high risk of losing jobs, even those marginal and menial jobs they can be expected to fill. Consequently, financial security and independence based on employment are described as precarious, and patients living under such conditions are portrayed as highly vulnerable. Conversely, patients receiving some form of entitlement assistance payment (e.g., Social Security, Supplemental Security Income, Social Security Disability Insurance, unemployment compensation) are considered more financially stable; their situations are described as more viable.

For example, in Metropolitan Court, David Jason testified that he paid the rent on a room in a "hotel" by washing dishes at a pizza parlor. He identified the restaurant by name, gave its address, and stated his employer's name. He said that his weekly income varied, but that he always made enough to pay the rent. In addition, Mr. Jason said he got free meals on each shift he worked. He indicated that he had been working at this particular restaurant for several months and had held similar positions for the past few years. The judge denied his writ, stating that Mr. Jason was gravely disabled: "I've got no guarantee that his financial needs will be met if I release him. . . . What if he loses the job?"

In contrast, in a preliminary report for Southern Court, Travis Roberts said he wanted to support himself by working as a house painter, but had lost a series of jobs over the past year, and was having difficulty finding another opportunity. He added, however, that he did receive veterans' disability payments each month. He was subsequently re-leased. In his explanation for not committing Mr. Roberts, the judge indicated that the veterans' benefits would be adequate to provide for Mr. Roberts's short-term needs. Note that in each case, testimony was produced that addressed the issue of basic necessities. The scenario that relied solely on gainful employment, however, was argued to be unten-able, while the one with a secure source of income (i.e., a monthly check from the government) was portrayed as viable.

During the entire course of this study, I never observed a judge release a patient whose claim of financial security and stability derived from his or her employment. However, attorneys and judges regularly cited in-come from Social Security or SSDI benefits as justification for returning persons to the community. Occasionally, being a registered welfare or AFDC recipient was noted as adequate grounds for release. Even com-plete financial dependency upon family members might be cited as a secure source of support because families are believed to be perma-nently responsible for their members.

Commitment hearings also focus on whether or not patients can dem-onstrate that they have secure housing arrangements that are not likely to be disrupted by disturbed or erratic behavior. It is often argued, for example, that persons who rent apartments on their own (even if they can document the ability to pay the rent being charged) are not as secure as persons living in a structured or institutionalized setting that was accustomed to dealing with the mentally ill, in a home they personally owned outright, a home owned by a family member, or even in a local Salvation Army or Rescue Mission dormitory. Two cases observed in Metropolitan Court illustrate some considerations that may be portrayed when discussing the viability of a patient's living arrangement.

Linda Golman, a thirty-five-year-old white female was taken to the county psychiatric facility from Metropolitan Airport, where she had created a disturbance on a shuttle bus. In court, a psychiatrist testified that she was gravely disabled, diagnosing her as bipolar disorder, manic type, accompanied by paranoid and grandiose delusions. The doctor noted that Ms. Golman had "no form of income, and no permanent address, no place to live." Ms. Golman, however, offered an alternative account, sometimes contradicting the doctor, sometimes offering expla-nations for the problematic circumstances the doctor described:

[6:3]   [Metropolitan Court; J1, DA1, PD4, Dr6, Linda Golman]

    PD4:   Would you like to leave the hospital?
     LG: Yes, of course.
    PD4:   Where would you go?

LG: I'd like to go to my old apartment. It's a mess though. ((silence)) Presently I've got a number of problems. I've been beaten and robbed. I need a criminal lawyer. I could have used a doctor. I guess right now I would have to stay with my mom.

PD4: What will you live on?

LG: I get SSI, but my check and my money were stolen. I have to get the old check cancelled, and get a new one issued. I get a check on the first of every month. I go to Mayfaire to pick it up.

PD4: Could you live in your apartment now?

LG: I could if I got it cleaned up. You see, the sewer overflowed. It's a basement apartment and it backed up and overflowed in my place. It wasn't my fault. (I've been good about paying my rent and I think the landlord would let me come back.) I guess if I've been tossed out, I'd have trouble getting back in, but I didn't do it. I may have to go to my mom's, but I don't want to be a burden to Mom. We haven't gotten along too well for a few years. I'd really rather live alone.

She continued to explain her financial circumstances under cross-examination:

[6:4] [Metropolitan Court; J1, DA1, PD4, Dr6, Linda Golman]

DA1: What were you doing at the airport?

LG: I was planning a trip, going overseas. I was going to go to Russia if I could. So I was at the airport, and I wanted to go out to lunch. So I took the bus to a hotel to eat. When I was done there, I got back on the bus, but while I was waiting there these three girls came up to me and hit me on the head. I got stabbed, and they must have took my money. They robbed me right there. That caused some commotion. (DA1 asks several questions seeking clarification of the details of this incident. LG responds to the questions.)

DA1: So you ended up without any money.

LG: That's right. They got it and my check.

DA1: And you can't go to your mother's, right?

LG: Well, we don't get along, but I don't want to be a burden. I'd be gone as soon as I got a place of my own.

Upon requestioning, the psychiatrist indicated that Ms. Golman's condition had improved greatly since entering the hospital and that the medication he prescribed for her was apparently working very well. Although he reiterated his opinion that she was still gravely disabled, he acknowledged that she was "just about ready to be released." The judge then asked what the hospital social worker could do to help Ms. Golman's financial and housing problems, and was told that the social worker could do nothing if Ms. Golman was released. The judge asked if Ms. Golman had relatives who would provide a place for Ms. Golman and was told that her mother did not think they could get along and refused to take Ms. Golman in. Finally, the judge questioned Ms. Golman at length, going over some questions the PD and DA had previously asked, adding some new ones of his own. Her responses seemed composed and rational.

Ultimately, the judge denied Ms. Golman's writ and ordered her commitment on the basis of grave disability for the remainder of her fourteen-day certification (nine days) with the following explanation:

[6:5] [Metropolitan Court; J1, DA1, PD4, Dr6, Linda Golman]

J1:

> The court notes that this woman is ready to leave the hospital—she seems to be doing just fine right now—and once she gets some money, the court will reconsider its decision. I'm very impressed with you [to Ms. Golman], but you just don't have any place to go. Out there like that you'll just get worse again. I'm finding you gravely disabled. You stay in the hospital for the next few days and then maybe you can set out on your own. Linda, you take care of yourself. I know you can do it. We'll keep you in just until you get yourself squared away.

In another case, Melvin Jackson, a thirty-five-year-old African American male, had been hospitalized by the police for wandering in the street in a very disheveled condition, babbling incoherently. He was diagnosed by the testifying psychiatrist as a chronic schizophrenic, undifferentiated type, and was reported to be quite delusional. The psychiatrist testified that Mr. Jackson had been evicted from his apartment, had lost contact with his wife, and had only six cents to his name when he was admitted to the hospital. He went on to say that Mr. Jackson claimed that he received five hundred dollars per month in disability payments, but the psychiatrist indicated that there was no evidence of this. Mr. Jackson, said the doctor, had been hospitalized eleven times in the past twelve years.

Mr. Jackson, however, testified that he had both plans and resources for living in the community.

[6:6] [Metropolitan Court; J1, DA4, PD6, Dr7, Melvin Jackson]

>PD6: If you are released, will you go to the [Rescue] Mission?
>MJ: Yes.
>PD6: Have you stayed there before?
>MJ: Yes, sir. They give you three meals a day. Then you work, do chores, and then the preacher comes and talks to you about God. They give you a room for the night. They give you a ticket for the room.
>PD6: Do you get a check each month?
>MJ: Yes, on the first of each month. Five hundred dollars Social Security.

PD6: Where do you get the check?

MJ: I pick it up at the office downtown on Spruce St. I get a check on the first. I got one on the first when I was living with my wife, but she got in a fight with some other tenant and we was evicted. If I got out now, I'd live in the Mission downtown.

Mr. Jackson repeated that he was no longer interested in living with his wife because "she causes me too much trouble." Later, under cross-examination, he recounted the details of losing his latest five-hundred-dollar check:

[6:7] [Metropolitan Court; J1, DA4, PD6, Dr7, Melvin Jackson]

DA4: What happened to all your money, the five hundred dollars?

MJ: I spent it in restaurants on food. And then, what I had left, a police ranger took it out of my pocket. Took thirty dollars.

DA4: A police ranger? Tell me about this. Tell me about someone taking your money.

MJ: I was on this bus going across Rosemont [a bad section of town]. I wouldn't walk those streets. When this fella in a uniform gets on. A police ranger. ((silence)) You know with one of those hats and a badge. He starts talking to people and then he's asking me where I'm going and why I'm not at home, all sorts of stuff. ((silence)) First he says I'm gonna be arrested but then he just reaches into my pocket and takes my money and says he'll forget it this time. He gets off the bus, but then at the next stop, he's right back on. This time he sees me, but before he can get me, I got out the back door.

J1: Did you report this?

MJ: Where? Who would I report it to? The cops? They did the taking.

J1: You're probably right.

In answer to further questions from the DA, Mr. Jackson said he did not think that he was seriously mentally ill, but would take medications if his doctor told him to. The judge then questioned Mr. Jackson, asking once again about his disability payments and where he received them, and rechecking the details of his plan to live at the mission. Finally, the judge granted the writ releasing Mr. Jackson, saying the following:

[6:8] [Metropolitan Court; J1, DA4, PD6, Dr7, Melvin Jackson]

J1:

In this case, I don't find evidence of grave disability. I believe Mr. Jackson can take care of himself, despite his serious problems, providing he goes to the mission, so I'm going to grant this writ. So you [Jackson] go to that mission and you stay there until August first [nine days hence] when you can go get your Social Security check and get your money and take up a respectable life. I'm granting this writ only provided you go to the mission and stay there. You know how to do that, you've done it before, and it sounds like a good place for you.

After the hearing, the judge reaffirmed his feeling that the mission was a good refuge for Jackson, no matter how bad his mental condition might get from time to time. "The place is familiar to him," the judge noted, "and they don't toss them out if they can't pay the rent. . . . He will be able to fit in there with the men's shelter program that they've got going."

In addition to illustrating the court's orientation to income and living situation, these cases suggest that arguments regarding material resources are not sufficient to establish that a patient's circumstances are tenable. Equally important are descriptions of how, and how effectively, a patient will be able to put those resources to use. Assuming patients are mentally ill leads court personnel to consider how apparently non-problematic, everyday situations might pose difficulties for psychiatrically disturbed persons. If a judge doubts a person's ability to negotiate transactions that are routine within the life-style that person plans to adopt, the judge will have difficulty justifying his or her release and commitment is likely. Patients must therefore argue that they have both access to resources and the ability to use them effectively.

Earning one's living through employment may be commendable, for example, but it can also be portrayed as a precarious situation for a mentally ill person who is likely to behave erratically and irresponsibly from time to time. Receiving a monthly check from a social service agency is considered a reliable source of income, but one must still demonstrate an ability to cash the check and spend the money wisely. Judges often argue that they prefer releasing persons into situations where their resources and affairs can be closely monitored, if not taken completely out of patients' hands, and where reliance upon patients' faculties is minimized.

Cases like those outlined above suggest that concerns about the mental condition of persons sought to be committed is less than paramount. The assumption of mental illness is crucial as background against which all evaluations are made, yet its independent effect on outcomes may be minor. (Chapter 7 will elaborate the importance of this assumption to the interpretive process.) Linda Golman, for example, was judged "ready to leave the hospital," implying that her psychiatric problems had abated. Still, her living situation was characterized as untenable, justifying the finding of grave disability. The judge argued that Ms. Golman had to be committed because she had no place to go. Melvin Jackson, on the other hand, was judged to have "serious problems" but his willingness to establish temporary domicile at the mission was cited as evidence of a tenable living situation, and grounds for release.

The Presence of Competent Caretakers

Commitment proceedings treated proposed living arrangements as one indicator of the extent to which those released had "support systems" within the community that could safeguard their welfare and contain their disruptive behavior. To this end, proceedings often focused on the presence or absence of someone who could "keep an eye" on the patient—a caretaker who would provide support and supervision. Indeed, at least two of the judges studied used the term *caretaker* to characterize persons whose cooperation in looking after the proposed patient might be enlisted. Such persons were typically portrayed as necessary components of a tenable living situation. Claims that a mentally ill person could adhere to prescribed conditions or regimens were viewed skeptically; proposals lacking close supervision were typically challenged. More acceptable arguments generally noted someone in the patient's vicinity—preferably a family member or other person living in close proximity to the person, like a board and care home manager— who would assume responsibility, at least informally, for supervising and checking up on the patient if she or he were released. Judges' explanations for their decisions often indicated that they expected released patients to be closely supervised so that when the "inevitable" relapse into disturbed behavior occurred, someone would be nearby to help contain it. If such a caretaker could not be established, judges argued, they were forced to continue hospitalization. As a Metropolitan Court judge noted in denying a writ (previously in extract [4:17]), "I don't see [the patient] being responsible for getting all the things he needs, and he doesn't have anyone who can do it for him."

Descriptions of a tenable living situation, then, are likely to include mentions of someone to "check up" on the person who is released to see if he or she is eating and sleeping regularly, maintaining reasonable personal hygiene, getting the proper medical care, and so on. Judges say they are more comfortable releasing persons whose financial matters are closely monitored (or, preferably, controlled) by a reliable person. All the courts studied regularly featured lines of questioning to determine who actually received the patient's income checks, and what was done with the money. Arguments that established that the checks went directly to some third party who would ration funds systematically or claims that the proposed patient regularly and promptly turned his or her check over to someone else were often cited as reasons for granting release.

For example, Hannah Smith, an elderly white female, was hospitalized because she had been giving away her money in public places. The police apprehended her when she caused a minor commotion trying to distribute dollar bills to patrons of a fast-food restaurant, clogging the service area and bringing business to a halt. According to the testifying psychiatrist, Mrs. Smith had been very agitated, confused, and incoherent at admission. His diagnosis was chronic bipolar disorder. During Mrs. Smith's testimony, the PD and the judge asked her a number of questions regarding her housing and financial arrangements. She indicated that she had a room and board arrangement with the owner of a private house: "I rent a very nice room and can use the kitchen any time I want. They fix meals. Three meals a day, or more if I want." She said her Social Security checks were sent directly to the home owner, who, after deducting her monthly payments, gave her the remainder of her money in weekly allotments. As for how she spent that money, she agreed that she had been giving it away: "I'll do anything I damn well please with my money."

The judge granted Mrs. Smith's writ, releasing her on the condition that she stay in contact with her son and daughter-in-law, and see her personal physician about her spells of agitation. His decision was accompanied by the following explanation:

[6:9]   [Metropolitan Court; J2, DA2, PD2, Dr10, Hannah Smith]

J2:

> This lady's neither dangerous or disabled. She seems to take care of herself for the most part. It looks like her landlord keeps an eye on her, makes sure she's all right. Her family has got to be willing to look in a little more often. . . . I don't like this money thing, but she does have a point. As long as the landlord gets his money first, and provides her with room and board, as long as she doesn't get her hands on the check first, she can't really do herself much harm. She can give away her money. It's her right. I may not think it's too smart, but that's not my business.

A wide range of persons is portrayed as potential caretakers, including family members, staff of board and care homes, physicians, landlords, neighbors, even the staff at the Salvation Army or Rescue Mission. Caretakers are entrusted with monitoring the patient's finances and day-to-day living habits, but tenability arguments often demand that caretakers assist released persons in obtaining some sort of treatment for their mental conditions as well. This might entail helping the person maintain an outpatient mental health care schedule or, more frequently, may involve monitoring the psychotropic medications that have nearly always been prescribed. By itself, the patient's promise to take medication was not a sufficiently compelling argument, so frequently pleas for release included a provision that a caretaker monitor medication compliance.

Commitment proceedings may focus on caretakers' competence as much as on patients'. In some instances—particularly in cases where dangerousness is a concern—caretakers may be challenged by describing them as physically incapable of enforcing desired behaviors or controlling the patient if the need arises. For example, a 6-foot 4-inch, 230-pound man, diagnosed as chronic paranoid schizophrenic, was judged gravely disabled because, the judge said, his elderly father and mother, who had agreed to take him in, could not control their son if his behavior got out of hand: "How are they going to manage this guy if he goes on some kind of rampage? He's just too big and strong for them." More easily controlled persons were not described as committable if they were going to be supervised by physically capable caretakers.

Concerns about circumstances and caretakers sometimes seem to overshadow those about the patient, particularly when the patient has "improved" or is "doing well" in the hospital. A judgment of grave disability is likely to be sustained, for example, if a caretaker is known to be unreliable, even if the patient seems relatively capable of living outside the hospital. In Metropolitan Court, for instance, Aron Cabel had been hospitalized after several episodes of unruly public behavior, and had been certified as both dangerous to others and gravely disabled. He said he had been off his medication when he experienced these episodes and promised to take them religiously in the future. Mr. Cabel said his wife had been helping with the medications, but recently she had been preoccupied with other things. Mr. Cabel claimed that his wife was responsible for the missed medications on the occasions that led to several of his disturbances. Most recently, he said, she forgot to bring his prescription on a cross-town trip. Mr. Cabel became unruly and was apprehended and hospitalized by the police.

The psychiatrist who examined Mr. Cabel indicated that Mr. Cabel seemed to do very well while on his medications, and that he had improved markedly while in the hospital. The judge denied Mr. Cabel's writ, explaining:

[6:10]   [Metropolitan Court, J2, DA4, PD1, Dr1, Aron Cabel]

J2:
> There have been a lot of incidents, getting into trouble. Too much to ignore here. . . . The doctor says you have improved, but you've still got the problem. . . . Without someone to see that you take your medicine, you'll be right back in. Better you should stay in where someone can help you, than to go back out with no help and have a relapse and undo all the good that's been done for you. We can't leave it up to your wife this time.

In this instance, the judge argued that the designated caretaker could not ensure that the patient would take his medications. The caretaker's inefficiency, the judge implied, rather than the patient's condition per se, was the crucial factor.

Cooperation with a Treatment Regime

Commitment proceedings also revolve around arguments concerning patients' cooperation with treatment for their alleged mental illness. As a Metropolitan Court judge noted, "They have to convince me that they will do as they are told, get the help they need, or I have to keep them in [the hospital]." Judges express this concern as they question patients, regularly focusing on patients' willingness to participate in outpatient treatment and, perhaps more importantly, to take prescribed psychotropic medication. DAs routinely argue that a patient's mental illness is "uncontrollable" or "not going to be adequately managed" if the person refuses to acknowledge the need for treatment. Such refusals are often cited as evidence of grave disability As another Metropolitan Court judge lectured to a person seeking release, "I'll continue to find you gravely disabled until you can recognize how important it is to get the help you need." Two cases from Metropolitan Court illustrate how patients' agreement or failure to cooperate with treatment are incorporated into commitment arguments.

Adolpho Arcelli was hospitalized for wandering the streets in what the police reported was "a disorganized state of mind." The testifying psychiatrist diagnosed him as chronic schizophrenic, disorganized type. Arcelli had been living with his father, receiving a monthly SSI check, and had seventy-nine dollars when he was hospitalized. His testimony was articulate and generally coherent, though on several occasions it became disorganized and difficult to comprehend. The PD asked Mr. Arcelli if he would consider living in a board and care facility. Mr. Arcelli said he preferred his own apartment, contending that he had been doing all right on his own. The PD then asked if he would agree to participate in a program of outpatient therapy, to which Mr. Arcelli replied, "There are two opinions on this" and proceeded on a rambling discussion of psychiatry and its utility. When the PD again asked if he would go to a community mental health center for therapy, Mr. Arcelli reluctantly agreed to "give it one try."

During cross examination, the DA asked Mr. Arcelli if he was mentally ill. Mr. Arcelli replied, "No." Had he ever been mentally ill? "No," he insisted again. Did he have any problems? "None," replied Mr. Arcelli. "Just collecting my SSI."

The judge tried, but could get no firmer commitment to outpatient therapy from Mr. Arcelli. Mr. Arcelli again refused to promise to take his medications. The judge finally began to lecture Mr. Arcelli on the necessity of getting help and being cooperative, concluding with the following:

[6:11]   [Metropolitan Court; J1, DA4, PD4, Dr12, Adolpho Arcelli]

J1:
   Will you give me your word you will take your medication? Will you go to outpatient therapy at the clinic? Will you give me your word? [Mr. Arcelli nods in reluctant agreement.] I want to get you somewhere where you will be watched out for and where you can get your medications, but you don't seem to want to cooperate. I just can't have that, so I'm denying the writ. At least in the hospital we can make sure you get the help that you need. . . . I find that Mr. Arcelli is gravely disabled.

In a contrasting case, Harry Rose, an African American about twenty years old had been hospitalized because his mother reported he was disruptive and delusional around the house. She said she would not take him back in the home "until he improves some," according to the testifying psychiatrist. Mr. Rose was diagnosed as having a reactive disorder.

Mr. Rose's testimony was very lucid and articulate. He said he had been delusional, but the delusions had disappeared. He argued that he could live with his father and sister if released. The PD asked Rose if he would seek outpatient treatment.

[6:12]   [Metropolitan Court; J1, DA1, PD3, Dr10, Harry Rose]

   HR: Yes, I'll do anything.
   J1:   How do we know you will?
   HR: I'll give you my word. My word is good.
   PD3: Do you have any problems?
   HR: Yes, a little here and there. I was supposed to go to the doctor for some pills, but when I didn't get them, I ended up in a crazy hospital.
   PD3: Have you been an outpatient before?
   HR: Yes.
   PD3: Will you go back to the treatment?
   HR: Yes, most definitely. I won't forget again.
   PD3: Will you take your medications?
   HR: Yes.
   J1:   Will you take it even if you feel you don't need it?
   HR: Yes, if the doctor said to. Anything he says.

The judge ruled that Mr. Rose was to be released if he could arrange for his father to come and get him: "As long as he's in treatment, I think this young man can go."

In both of these cases, the patients were well comported and articulate. Since most aspects of tenable community living circumstances were said to be in place, arguments concerning the patients' willingness to cooperate with ongoing treatment became central. Mr. Arcelli was reluctant to cooperate with a treatment regime and take his medications, factors the judge cited as he explained his decision to commit. Mr. Rose, however, was willing (indeed, he seemed almost eager) to agree to the judge's "treatment plan." By earnestly demonstrating his willingness to cooperate in getting the help the judge felt he needed, Mr. Rose offered the judge reasonable grounds for deciding upon release, factors he highlighted in his final ruling.[2]

Placing Insanity: Matching Needs to Accommodations

In a sense, commitment hearings attempt to minimize the harmful impact of persons thought to be mentally ill. Commitment decisions cannot simply be justified by arguments that a person is mentally disturbed, or that he or she is unable to care for him- or herself. Rather, judges typically point out the inability of the person's living situation to compensate for and contain the person's incapacities and disruptions. Arguments for and against commitment are formulated in highly contextual and specific terms, with reference to the patient both as a "social type"—one who is chronically mentally ill—and as a particular, locally situated individual who may or may not possess certain social skills and resources. Participants in commitment proceedings engage in practical reasoning about both the nature and consequences of mental illness and the salient features of community living arrangements for the released patient. They typify patients as chronic "crazy persons" in need of help, and project for them a set of traits and problems characteristic of this sort of person. The psychiatric details of a case are consequential only in the ways that they are made relevant to discussions of how patients conduct the routine and necessary transactions of daily life. Similarly, they typify living circumstances in terms of their ability to contain and control mentally ill persons.

Thus commitment decisions are not just about people and their psychiatric conditions. Nor are they simply about the relative advantages of institutional or community care. Rather, they are about fitting people to places. Throughout the commitment process, we hear that insanity must be properly placed to control its havoc. As a practical matter, tenable living circumstances are established in terms of the fit between the particular *needs* and *demands* of the patient in question and the *accommodations* available in a proposed living situation. The adequacy of a proposed living situation's accommodations can be interpreted only in light of its proposed occupant's needs and demands. A tenable situation is one that matches a patient's needs and demands with a living situation that satisfies those needs.

Consider how arguments for release in the cases outlined above all attempted to match the patients' needs with the accommodations available to them. The counterarguments detailed the ways in which the available community living arrangements were not suitably matched to these needs and demands, and how the hospital would better suit the persons involved. Patients were variously described as dangerous or docile, vulnerable or able to look out for themselves, manageable or uncooperative. And living arrangements were portrayed as varying with respect to their ability to provide for and adjust to the special needs that were cited. Particular circumstances, it was argued, might be appropriate for some people, and not for others. Living at the Rescue Mission, for example, was portrayed as a reasonable option for a middle-aged, indigent black man, but would not be considered appropriate for a woman or older person.

Accomplishing Tenability

Achieving tenability, then, involves arguments about how living situations might accommodate the needs and demands of the mentally ill. The discourse of commitment proceedings suggests the logic of a matching procedure whereby the patient and his or her proposed living situation are aligned and the suitability of one for the other is assessed. This decision logic was evident, for example, when the Metropolitan Court judge concluded that Melvin Jackson could be safely released to reside at the Rescue Mission because "he will be able to fit in there with the men's shelter program that they've got going." In essence, the judge argued that the situation was a suitable match to Jackson's special needs; the person fit the situation. In a sense, tenability amounts to the practical, descriptive conflation of persons and their situational accommodations.

The commonsense understanding of the decision-making process as a matching operation, however, glosses over the *accomplished* character of matches between persons and environments. It treats persons, situations, and the fit between the two as objective conditions that are uncovered and reported as part of commitment proceedings. My observations suggest, however, that descriptions of patients and assessments of living arrangements are situationally and rhetorically assembled; similarly, the match between them is an occasioned production. Court personnel actively seek out and invoke information that might be incorporated into tenability-related arguments, and speculate about the possible circumstances that might be arranged to accommodate released patients. They justify their arguments for and against commitment by strategically articulating patients' needs and attributes with the specific accommodations said to be available in (or absent from) proposed living situations. The "fit" between the two is therefore a product of participants' interpretive, descriptive activity. Whereas, on the surface, the decision-making process may resemble a *search* for and contingent *discovery* of a match between person and environment, that match or mismatch is better construed analytically as a rhetorical *accomplishment*.

Tenability or untenability is constructed, argued, contested, and negotiated. The salient aspects of patients' traits, conditions, and living circumstances emerge interactionally from within the commitment process itself. Myriad factors may coalesce in tenability assessments, but each must be made consequential by participants as they assemble the specifics of the case at hand. The relevance of any particular factor—psychiatric symptoms, behavioral tendencies, or situational contingencies—is not found in the person or situation per se. Rather, it emerges through commitment hearing discourse.

If we analyze commitment decision-making in terms of relations between fixed variables, we end up treating the variable components of tenability as if they were, in fact, both objective features of a case and consequential for that case. Doing so overlooks participants' authorship of the artfully structured logical connections and consistencies that warrant their arguments and decisions. But if we acknowledge that participants create, rather than discover, person-situation matches and mismatches, we abandon the conception of participants as mere "computerized dopes" (Maynard 1984)—that is, passive information processors. Instead, we view them as strategically astute tacticians who construct rather than respond to the consistencies and inconsistencies that their accounts reveal. Participants knowledgeably and intentionally formulate and manipulate person-environment scenarios as rhetorical maneuvers supporting particular dispositions of the case at hand.

Because of this, commitment decisions are not easily predicted from mere knowledge of abstract variables and relations between them. Matches between persons and situational accommodations are not found in the concrete "data" of case-relevant information; they are manufactured in case-relevant discourse. As Emerson's (1989) analysis of psychiatric emergency teams suggests, participants in the commitment process actively create or deny situations' tenability. They select and elaborate the relevant factors, reflexively producing the conditions that their acts of inquiry and argument ostensibly only discover and report.

Research seeking to explain commitment proceedings by reference to relations between fixed variables is all but insensitive to the locally emergent character of tenability-related factors. Findings derived from a fixed-variable approach should thus be held in dubious regard. Indeed, many of the inconsistent, equivocal, or inconclusive research findings regarding commitment proceedings may be due to researchers' insistence on conceptualizing the commitment process in terms of fixed variables rather than interpretive practices.

Tenability and Accountability

In one respect, the preceding analysis focuses on tenability as the basis for justifying commitment arguments and decisions. But it also says something more about interpretive and decision-making practices than how they are justified. Organizations and institutions—like commitment proceedings—can be construed as "quasi-boundaried" frameworks of accounting practices (Heritage 1983). They are domains within which actions and actors are constitutively defined and evaluated by reference to circumscribed vocabularies of accounts. Normative standards of accountability supply a "grid" through which actions are understood and assessed. Accountability frameworks thus represent institutionalized, normal, typical features of the domain of action in question (Heritage 1983). Conduct—regardless of its objectives—will tend to be designed and shaped in response to constraints imposed by this frame. Anticipation of demands for accountability helps organize and channel actions to keep them locally justifiable.

Commitment arguments and decisions are assembled so that they appear to be legally, psychiatrically, and practically justifiable. The orientation to tenability respects the configuration of a locally relevant accountability framework that embodies these concerns. The assumption of patients' mental illness, while relegated to the background, is never forgotten as the limitations and problems of the mentally ill are constantly used to frame tenability assessments. The practical matter of managing potential havoc is invariably central. And the legality of arguments and decisions is constantly displayed in the ways that descriptions are linked to legally relevant categories and arguments are legally framed and articulated.

Hearing participants, then, routinely use the language of the law in conjunction with practical concerns for managing troubled and troublesome persons in order to provide their accounts and explanations with the appearance of being reasoned, orderly, principled, warranted, legal, and practical. Arguments and decisions are justified by displaying how they comply with, or are compelled by, the need to contain the havoc of mental illness under the aegis of the law. Tenability constructions both reflect and respect the local framework of legal and practical accountability.

* * * * *

Tenability concerns emphasize situational factors, seemingly minimizing the importance of psychiatric considerations. Chapter 7 reasserts the significance of mental illness for commitment decisions, showing how the assumption that patients are severely disturbed serves as an interpretive framework within which tenability is accomplished.

Notes

1.   Warren (1977) argues that considerations of a person's ability to function within the mental health system are more relevant for commitment decisions than are considerations of patients' lives or proposed lives in the community. My observations suggest that information regarding behavior while hospitalized is used to project future behavior patterns for persons whose release is being considered. In-hospital behavior is routinely cited as grounds for further hospitalization, with the suggestion that a patient who cannot function within a sheltered environment will do even worse on the outside. Ironically, doing well in the hospital does not assure release; occasionally a patient's successful adaptation to hospital life is argued as grounds for continued hospitalization, "because he is doing so well."

2.   Harry Rose had been in the audience during the Arcelli hearing. His conduct during his own hearing suggests that he may have learned something about how to argue for his own release as well as how to comport himself to display a willingness to cooperate.

Chapter 7

Mental Illness Assumptions

Framing tenability as the foremost consideration seemingly de-emphasizes the role that mental illness and psychiatric assessments play in the commitment process. Clearly, the popular stereotype that commitment is based predominantly on psychiatric factors is erroneous, but it would be mistaken to suggest that commitment proceedings are indifferent to the mental condition of those for whom commitment is considered. The law requires the demonstration of serious mental illness, and we have seen the extent to which hearing participants are concerned with patients' interactional competence. But equally important are the myriad ways that assumptions about patients' mental illnesses serve as interpretive frameworks for evaluating individuals' prospects for successfully living in circumstances outside the psychiatric ward (Holstein 1987b).[1] Assessments of patients' mental condition and appraisals of their competence and/or dangerousness are *reflexively* related so that each is practically established only in light of the other. Relating assumptions about patients' mental illness to their particular material and social circumstances is a central interpretive procedure in commitment proceedings.

Mental Illness Assumptions as Interpretive Schemes

While mental illness is not sufficient grounds for hospitalization, its assumption profoundly influences how commitment cases are argued and interpreted. Most importantly, perhaps, imputations of psychiatric disorder provide a distinctive and immutable background against which all other assessments and evaluations are made. Mental illness thus serves as a scheme of interpretation (Schutz 1962) that imposes a particular context upon all other information regarding the patient, embedding knowledge of and judgments about the person and his or her behavior

133

in a distinctive body of commonsense knowledge about mentally ill persons.

As court personnel impute mental illness, they implicitly structure their interpretations of patients' behavior more generally. That behavior, viewed as a product of mental illness, then serves to further document the presence of the illness itself. Thus, descriptions of patients as mentally ill and subsequent interpretations of their behavior stand in a fundamentally dialectical relation to one another. The underlying pattern— mental illness—provides the basis for interpreting actions in a meaningful, distinctive way. The actions, so interpreted, in turn serve to document, substantiate, and sustain the underlying pattern (Garfinkel 1967).

The Metropolitan Court hearing involving Philip Walters, a twenty-five-year-old white male illustrates how the mental illness assumption reflexively shapes and is shaped by interpretations of patients' actions. Walters was alleged to be gravely disabled, and through examination of the psychiatrist and cross-examination of Mr. Walters himself, the DA tried to show that Mr. Walters was incapable of providing for his basic necessities because his illness rendered him incapable of managing his money. At the end of the hearing, the judge asked Mr. Walters just how he intended to support himself if he was released. Mr. Walters indicated that he would cash his veterans' benefits check and use the money to pay his rent. The judge then asked what he would do with the remaining funds, to which Mr. Walters replied, "I'd spend it on food and clothes, and what's left on girls." Later, in his explanation for continuing Mr. Walters's hospitalization, the judge noted the following:

[7:1]   [Metropolitan Court; J1, DA3, PD2, Dr9, Philip Walters]

J1:
> Mr. Walters's ability to manage his finances appears to be impaired. His plans for spending money are inappropriate. . . . He's in no position to be throwing his money away on women. It's a pretty clear sign that he's not really well yet.

The assumed underlying pattern—that Mr. Walters was a mentally ill person—provides the interpretive resources necessary to portray Mr. Walters's use of his money for "girls" as irresponsible behavior. Attributed to a "normal" twenty-five-year-old male, this statement is unremarkable, a typical pursuit for someone of that type. But within the mental illness schema, it can be described as "inappropriate" behavior, a "clear sign" of mental illness. Mr. Walters's claim is rendered inappropriate when attached to the underlying pattern. At the same time, the inappropriate claim serves as a document of the pattern itself. Document and pattern are thus mutually constitutive.

In light of the mental illness assumption, nearly any problematic or unconventional behavior—and much behavior that might be considered normal or routine for others—is readily construed as bizarre, crazy, or symptomatic. Practicing the piano can be characterized as a "music obsession"; wearing a different scarf each day of the week can be portrayed as "obsessive fetishism." In a case involving a patient named Richard Owen, what might otherwise be described as avid religiosity was interpreted as a disabling obsession. Mr. Owen, a middle-aged white male, had been hospitalized at his brother's request for not eating or sleeping for several days. The brother said that Mr. Owen had been acting in a bizarre fashion and had made "looking for signs of Jesus" his sole pastime. At the hearing, Mr. Owen claimed that he had no problems eating or sleeping, indicating that he had not missed a day at work and felt fine. Regarding religious matters, Mr. Owen said he had recently heard a radio evangelist discussing signs of the second coming of Jesus Christ that could be found both in scripture and in historical and recent events. Mr. Owen said he was interested in verifying these signs and had set out to do his own research using the Bible, history books, encyclopedias, and other reference materials. He said that he may have recently become somewhat "obsessed, if that means working on it a lot." For the past week, he claimed he had been coming straight home from work to pursue the project, not taking time out for meals, but eating snacks when he got hungry as he worked through the night trying to complete his study by the end of the week.

On the night of his hospitalization, Mr. Owen said he left his home for about an hour to go to the store, and upon his return found all his papers strewn about his apartment. He said he called his brother, who lived nearby, to see if he had any idea what might have happened, and in the course of their discussion, described the research he had been doing. Mr. Owen then testified to the following admission:

[7:2]   [Metropolitan Court; J2, DA4, PD1, Dr21, Richard Owen]

RO:

> I know I shouldn't have said this, or at least not put it this way, but I told him [his brother], maybe this is another sign from God. Maybe it was done by angels. I shouldn't have said that. I was just talking. I was frightened. It was a nightmare. I'm giving up looking for signs now, though. I've finished my study.

The judge ordered Mr. Owen's commitment, stating that Mr. Owen had "debilitating psychological problems" that rendered him gravely disabled. He referred to Mr. Owen's mental illness as a basis for what he called Mr. Owen's "obsession with the spiritual world." Mr. Owen, he said, was "showing the kind of extreme behavior that's not unusual for sick people like him. They sometimes forget to take care of themselves." The judge thus used mental illness as an interpretive resource for making sense of Mr. Owen's behavior.

Commitment decisions are always made within the context and use the interpretive resources that the assumption of mental illness provides. Patients and their conduct are portrayed and assessed against this background so that anything said or done is viewed as the claim or behavior of a "crazy person." Cast in this light, their testimony and behavior are always suspect. Their credibility is constantly challenged and their claimed capabilities discounted. Behavior that might pass for normal or competent is regarded as atypical, artificial, or transitory. And, of special consequence, the assumption fundamentally shapes arguments regarding the tenability of living situations. A situation's tenability is not formulated as it would be for a "normal" person; the arrangement's viability must be established for a very special sort of person—one who is mentally disturbed and has a very special set of problems and needs.[2]

Mental Illness and Credibility

The mental illness assumption consistently undermines patients' credibility. One Metropolitan Court judge described his perspective in the following way, suggesting that he was skeptical of anything a patient might say:

[7:3]   [Metropolitan Court; J1]

> You have to be very careful about what you believe and what you don't. It's not that they're lying. They just don't know what the truth is. They aren't too keen on reality, if you know what I mean.

Of course, this handicaps patients when they are called upon to testify because all their accounts and explanations are suspect. Other participants are unlikely to treat patients' claims as completely viable as they formulate their own accounts and arguments They are reluctant to rely upon claims made by "crazy" people, claims that cannot be trusted or believed. Even patients' statements regarding factual information are more likely to be disbelieved, suspected, or discounted than statements made by other witnesses.

Patient Harris Charles, for example, indicated under cross-examination that he lived in the "Marriott Plaza" hotel. He said that a friend had paid his rent for the past few months. When asked the friend's name, Mr. Charles declined to reveal it, claiming that his friend was a "philanthropist" who wanted to remain anonymous: "He doesn't want to be exposed to all those people who would be begging for his help." In explaining his subsequent finding of grave disability, the judge noted that Mr. Charles would benefit from hospitalization because "he has no place to stay on a consistent basis." This account completely disregarded Mr. Charles's testimony regarding his place of residence and source of support. Perhaps his claim was problematic, but it was treated as if it was certainly untrue, apparently because it was the account of a deranged person. "That story about the hotel and the philanthropist was just too crazy," the judge explained later. The judge contended he had no reason to believe such a "wild story":

[7:4]   [Metropolitan Court; J2]

> There's no way in the world a guy like that could live there. If that's the best story he can come up with, I've got to assume he's got no place to go. The psychiatrist says the same thing. It's a fabrication of a disturbed mind.

The assumption of mental illness makes it possible to resolve conflicting testimony by framing it as a choice between the claims of a "sane" person (who is frequently a psychiatric professional) or those of a "madman" or "crazy person."

The manner in which Mr. Charles's testimony was discounted reveals another subtle consequence of the assumption of psychiatric disorder. Rather than viewing Mr. Charles's claim as a *report*—albeit fraudulent— about his place of residence, the testimony was framed as a *symptom* of Mr. Charles's illness, "a fabrication of a disturbed mind." This practical distinction between report and symptom casts patients' talk and behavior as outward signs of their "known" underlying trouble. In this case, what might otherwise pass for rationally motivated, but possibly deceitful, description (that is, the claim to reside in an expensive hotel) was portrayed as a sign of mental illness. Taken to the extreme, any claim of "normalcy" or "mental health" made by a patient might be described as a symptom rather than a report, and thus be discounted because it reveals the patient's failure to comprehend and acknowledge the fact of his or her illness. Not recognizing the illness, it might be argued, is clearly symptomatic of that very illness.

This situation is not unlike circumstances mental patients encounter elsewhere in the mental health care delivery system. For example, research amply documents the extent to which mental patients' claims are routinely discounted in a variety of treatment settings (Goffman 1961; Rosenhan 1973). A significant difference here is that this is a legal setting, in which matters of fact are to be impartially and concretely established. All witnesses, including patients, are sworn to tell the truth, yet it is consistently argued that patients are incapable of valid testimony. Conventions of the legal system are loosely observed for everyone else, but it is assumed that patients cannot honor the oath they take. But their assumed misrepresentation of the facts is not punished through contempt citations—as one presumably should be punished for lying while under oath—because such false claims are treated as symptoms of illness, not rationally calculated deceit or lies. So, while patients' testimony may be discounted, their assumed mental illness does protect them from accusations of willfully violating legal constraints.

Contextualizing Patients' Performance

Not only is the assumption of mental illness used to discredit patients' testimony, but court personnel also voice doubts concerning patients' courtroom demeanor, comportment, and self-presentation. Court personnel go beyond the mere content of official testimony, citing other aspects of observable courtroom behavior as relevant decision-making data. Thus, how the patient comports him- or herself, how he or she responds to questioning and conducts him- or herself while being examined by counsel, and even how he or she acts when not directly involved in the courtroom proceedings may be incorporated into commitment arguments. In a sense, patients are "on trial" the entire day in court, not just the few minutes spent on the witness stand, and are seldom "off stage." Any observable behavior can be referenced as an indication of their mental or interactional competence.

"Reality Checks" and Practical Performance

Court personnel try to use firsthand evidence in their arguments about how well patients might respond to the demands of community living. An Eastern Court judge, for example, indicated that he thought that formal courtroom hearings were essential to the commitment process, not just for legal reasons, but because they provided the opportunity to "check out" and "test" the patient's ability to function outside the sheltered world of the mental hospital or community mental health center. "We give them a chance to prove themselves," he noted, "by letting them defend themselves. If they can't manage to show me that they can handle themselves, then I'm not gonna release them."

Some of the testing appears to be checks on "reality orientation," a practice argued to be common in civil commitment proceedings (Scheff 1964; Warren 1982). This was apparently the case in Metropolitan Court, where judges repeatedly asked questions that demanded factual information from the patient like: What day is it? Where are you right now? How do you get to your mother's house from Southpark? What is fifty plus thirty-five? Consider, for example, the following series of questions that the judge asked Regina Farmer after the DA had completed his cross-examination:

[7:5]   [Metropolitan Court; J2, DA1, PD3, Dr2, Regina Farmer]

1.	J2:	I'd like to ask a few questions if I might. ((silence)) Is that
2.		OK with you?
3.	RF:	Sure.
4.	J2:	What is your full name?
5.	RF:	Regina Victoria Farmer.
6.	J2:	Where do you live?
7.	RF:	My mother's house is at 3890 Benson.
8.	J2:	What is your phone number?
9.	RF:	5 5 5 8 6 4 2.
10.	J2:	What is your grandmother's phone number?
11.	RF:	That's 5 5 5 6 7 9 3.
12.	J2:	What's your grandmother's name, Regina?
13.	RF:	Estelle Crawford.
14.	J2:	Who are what are the names of some of your other relatives who
15.		live in the area?
16.	RF:	My aunt's name is Josephine Williams, and my cousin Janette
17.		lives with her. ((silence)) You want more?
18.	J2:	No that's fine. Do you know what day it is today?
19.	RF:	Thursday.
20.	J2:	And do you know where you are right now?
21.	RF:	Well I'm in court, Metropolitan Court. ((silence)) I think
22.		we're down on San Duarte Road somewhere.
23.	J2:	Could you get home from here?
24.	RF:	I said I figure I could get a bus if you showed me where it
25.		stopped.
26.	J2:	How're you going to do that? Do you know about riding the bus?
27.	RF:	I've done it plenty. You just ask the driver.

In many respects, the series resembles a reality check, with the questions embedded from lines 4 through 26 inquiring into the patient's ability to relate the facts of the circumstances surrounding her. Questions on lines 18 and 20 are classic in this regard. But as the sequence progresses, its practical orientation also becomes apparent. It is evident that many of these questions were not asked to evaluate the patient's reality orientation as much as they were intended to provide documents of her current ability to locate herself in the community, proceed to intended destinations, and conduct the routine transactions of everyday life that release into the community would demand. These may be conceived as very practical questions, their importance deriving from a mundane or literal interpretation of their significance. Correct answers document a sort of competence in community living; incorrect responses provide the basis for arguing that the person would have difficulty negotiating life outside an institution (but not necessarily a faulty grasp of "reality"). For example, at line 20, the inquiry "Do you know where you are right now?" and its answer have very real practical consequences if Ms. Farmer is going to be released, as the following questions (lines 23 and 26) reveal.

Causal attributions are integral features of judges' accounts for commitment decisions, and the presumption of patients' mental illness supports the notion that the cause of any displayed incompetence be located *within* the patient. An incorrect answer will be cited as a symptom, both a product and a document of a disturbed mind; other possible reasons for a wrong answer are usually ignored. For example, a Metropolitan Court judge refused to consider the possibility that Jefferson Smith's inability to state his mother's address might be due to his recent arrival in town, or his recent ten-day hospitalization where he was heavily medicated, or even his nervousness about appearing in court—all possible explanations suggested by Smith's attorney. Instead the judge agreed:

[7:6]   [Metropolitan Court; J2, DA1, PD1, Dr14, Jefferson Smith]

J2:

> This man's mental condition interferes with his ability to do the day-to-day functions that he has to do if he wants to live with his family. His psychosis has impaired his memory. . . . He's lost. He can't look out for himself.

The assumption that Mr. Smith was mentally ill precludes assigning other causes (including simple ignorance) for his misstatement of the address. Thus, those situational explanations that relieve the "normal" actor from responsibility for many minor transgressions in the course of everyday life are invalid when evaluating the meaning of a "mentally ill" person's mistakes. The assumption of mental illness implies that good cause for perceived incompetence can be found in the patient's "sick" mind. External causes need not be seriously considered.

Despite assuming that persons sought to be committed are mentally disturbed, court personnel contend that most patients are conscious of their courtroom demeanor. "Let's face it," noted an Eastern Court judge, "they're on their best behavior. They're doing everything they can to hide their condition." Patients are portrayed as intentionally concealing or restraining symptoms that lurk just below any facade of normalcy that may be temporarily sustained. Composed, situationally appropriate demeanor and organized, articulate testimony are often discounted, if not disregarded, as valid indicators of patients' capabilities; they are said to be little more than "acting" or "performances," contrived self-presentations that quickly evaporate once the patient lets down his or her guard. Conversely, any behavior that might be interpreted as symptomatic of mental illness is readily cited as evidence of the patient's true condition. Indeed, any "slip-up" may be described as the mere "tip of the iceberg" of deranged behavior that can be caused by mental illness.

Medication and Performance

The fact that most involuntary commitment hearings are held while patients are undergoing evaluation and treatment further influences interpretations of what these persons say and do. Most patients are receiving psychotropic medications at the time of their hearings. While court personnel do not believe such medications cure mental illness, they do say they can be effective in containing or suppressing symptoms. Whatever rational, composed, "appropriate" behavior patients might display, then, is often attributed to their medications. And because they are assumed to be mentally ill and mental illness is assumed to have visible symptoms, any absence of symptoms is attributed to the drugs, as one judge noted:

[7:7] [Metropolitan Court; J1]

> These people are very, very sick. And without their medications they don't stand a chance. Usually the medications give them a chance to pull themselves together, get things under control. But they need to stay on them. It's the only way they can maintain. This last fellow today seemed very together, but take him off meds and he's in his own world again. He can do just fine—like today—if he'll just take his meds.

Thus, patients are held responsible for all "inappropriate" behavior, but "appropriate" or "competent" behavior may be attributed to medications. If one is believed to be mentally ill, but on medication, one's personal competence is continually questioned; even the absence of symptoms is attributed to medication and thus may be cited as evidence of the need for commitment.

The assumption of mental illness is virtually self-sustaining as it promotes interpretations that further document mental illness's presence. Harris Charles's claim of living in the "Marriott Plaza," for example, was claimed to be a "fabrication of a disturbed mind." This fabrication was later cited as evidence of Mr. Charles's mental illness, reflexively reifying the very assumption that cast the claim as fabrication. In another case, patient Marie Albeck testified in an articulate and rational manner, giving every indication of interactional competence, even by the admission of the judge who ruled her gravely disabled. Yet the DA argued that her composed demeanor was ephemeral, merely a temporary departure from, or disguise for, the chaotic behavior of the mentally ill person she was "known" to be. Denying her writ, the judge added, "She's really disturbed, but she doesn't always show it. She's so sick that she tries to hide her illness even when people just want to help her. We know it can't last." Even her "good behavior"—interpreted as a calculated yet pathological departure from the typical—was used to document her mental disturbance. Once assumed, mental illness remains an almost incorrigible description of persons whose commitment is under consideration.

Suspending the Assumption

There are, of course, instances when patients' testimony or performances are not simply discounted because of their assumed mental illness. Some of these cases involve what participants interpret as extraordinary displays of competence by the patient. Others occur when court personnel can argue that there has been a violation of organizational procedure or expectation, thus undermining the mental illness assumption. For example, on rare occasions in Metropolitan Court, psychiatrists or private attorneys who are inexperienced with commitment procedures may seek hospitalization in violation of either explicit or implicit commitment criteria. They may argue, for example, that less restrictive treatment alternatives need not be considered because of some special circumstance relating to the patient—usually the clear evidence of severe mental disorder. If other court personnel are not convinced, all assumptions about the background features of the case and the patient may be suspended. Thus, the assumption that alternative remedies have already been attempted will not hold, and the usual attribution of mental illness may be tentative or problematic. The patient's testimony and behavior may then be interpreted against a new background, through a different interpretive framework.

Consider the case of Janet Conrow, a twenty-two-year-old white female whose family had engaged a psychiatrist in private practice, Dr. Ryan, to help involuntarily hospitalize her. According to her family, Ms. Conrow had been very depressed, then had become delusional and agitated. In response to commands "from inside her head," Ms. Conrow had tried to kill the family dog and threatened some neighborhood children. The family also claimed that Ms. Conrow had repeatedly been uncontrollable in public places and finally had to be physically removed from a local shopping mall and transported to a psychiatric facility by the police at the parents' request. She had been held there over the weekend, and after a psychiatric evaluation, the parents asked Dr. Ryan to pursue involuntary hospitalization because Ms. Conrow refused to stay in the hospital voluntarily.

At the hearing, which was his first in Metropolitan Court, Dr. Ryan sought Ms. Conrow's involuntary commitment, arguing that he had diagnosed her as schizophrenic and that she was gravely disabled as well as dangerous to herself and others. After seeking some clarifications regarding Dr. Ryan's recommendation, the judge asked how long Ms. Conrow had been under Dr. Ryan's care and what her history of outpatient psychiatric treatment had been. He was somewhat surprised to hear that Dr. Ryan had been brought onto the case only recently and that Ms. Conrow had no treatment history. She had previously seen the Conrow family physician to discuss her feelings of "agitation," but he had done nothing more than prescribe a mild sedative. At this point, the judge launched a rather extended lecture on the mandate of community mental health care, then aggressively requestioned Dr. Ryan regarding his recommendation to commit when alternatives had not been explored. Dr. Ryan reiterated his belief that Ms. Conrow's symptoms were so bad and her behavior so bizarre and uncontrollable that institutional control and monitoring was clearly indicated, especially in light of her parents' request.

When she testified, Ms. Conrow was agitated, but coherent. She admitted to hearing voices, but claimed that she was not going to listen to them in the future. She repeatedly denied the need for psychiatric care, but acknowledged that she could use some help "to make her feel better." The judge asked her if she would be willing to see a "counsellor" at a community mental health center, if she would agree to take medications, and if she would move in with her parents "until she was feeling like herself again." She reluctantly agreed to all three stipulations, although she claimed she did not want to live at home and continued to assert that she was not the only one who needed help: "This whole mess is crazy. I'll go to the shrink if you say so, but why are you just picking on me?"

The judge released Janet Conrow with the following explanation:

[7:8] [Metropolitan Court; J1, DA5, PD7, Dr25, Janet Conrow]

J1:

> This woman obviously needs help, but I think she can get it without hospitalizing her at this time. She says she can keep her act together on her own, so I'll trust her to keep her promise to get the kind of care she needs and give her a chance. . . . If this doesn't work out, we can always bring you back here, young lady. Let's not let your emotional problems get out of hand. You get help, so we don't have to force it on you.

Later, the judge indicated that he was ambivalent about releasing a woman whose family sought her hospitalization, but felt there was insufficient evidence to warrant Ms. Conrow's commitment: "She's got troubles, no doubt about that, but it's not clear that she can't overcome them. Sometimes we have to find out if they can really manage or not."

Janet Conrow's case was uncharacteristic because a violation of the court's expectation of prior processing dislodged the typical interpretive framework through which patients are portrayed. The judge could not fully sustain the assumption that Ms. Conrow was mentally ill and disabled because he could not reference a typical organizational and remedial history. Consequently, he was willing to honor her claims to a much greater extent than usual. Indeed, the judge directly incorporated her promises regarding how she would manage her life in the community into his explanation for his decision.

Typical assumptions about patients may thus become problematic if features of the case at hand cannot be articulated with the "normal case." When assumptions are altered, the ensuing formulations of matters at hand may change, as might the commitment decision and its justificatory accounts.

Tenability and Mental Illness

As Chapter 6 suggests, commitment proceedings also focus on the tenability of a patient's proposed community living circumstances. As a practical matter, however, tenability must be established *for a mentally ill person*. In their courtroom presentations and interpretations, court personnel argue that a tenable living situation is one that accommodates, contains, and controls the havoc that is assumed to accompany mental illness. Consequently, they consider the situation and its occupants' ability to deal with instability, vulnerability, irresponsibility, dangerousness, and erratic or bizarre behavior, even if the patient in question has given no concrete evidence of possessing these traits.

As noted above, when presented in light of the assumption of mental illness, patients' claims regarding viable living arrangements are regarded with suspicion. The practicalities of how patients will support themselves are always a concern because it is assumed that mental illness renders its victims so unstable, unreliable, and incompetent that they are incapable of making and managing money. Because the mentally ill behave erratically, judges and DAs frequently argue that patients are likely to lose even those marginal and menial jobs that they are most likely to get. Consequently, financial support based on employment is portrayed as highly vulnerable, and living arrangements dependent upon holding a job are described as clearly untenable. Conversely, patients who claim to support themselves on some sort of entitlement assistance (e.g., Social Security, Supplemental Security Income, Social Security Disability Insurance, unemployment compensation, veterans' benefits) are described as more financially stable; their living situations are considered more viable.

Consider the Eastern Court case involving Ned Yost, a twenty-seven-year-old white male who had been hospitalized after being arrested for causing a public disturbance in an all-night doughnut shop. At his commitment hearing, Mr. Yost testified that he had been supporting himself by working as a busboy. The restaurant had agreed to participate in a locally sponsored vocational rehabilitation program and hired Mr. Yost upon his completion of the program's job training. Mr. Yost gave the judge the name and address of the restaurant and said that his supervisor could be called to verify his employment. Mr. Yost indicated that he had the job for almost three months and previously held several jobs of this nature. He was making the minimum wage, but was working enough hours to earn over one hundred dollars weekly, after taxes. This was enough to live on, he claimed, because he only paid $276 a month for rent and received free meals on the job.

At the hearing, no attempt was made to contact Mr. Yost's employer or anyone from the vocational rehabilitation program. Mr. Yost was committed, with the explanation that his financial situation was too precarious to be considered viable. The judge argued:

[7:9] [Eastern Court; J1, DA1, PD2, Dr1, Ned Yost]

J1:

> The option of living outside [the hospital] at the present time isn't very realistic. He is in no condition to fend for himself, support himself. If I release Mr. Yost, he will surely lose his job, just go out and do something to get fired. His behavior is too unpredictable. And when he loses the job, where will he be? Nowhere. I just can't release him to face that prospect. He's better off getting the help he needs in the hospital.

The assumption of Mr. Yost's mental illness seemingly made it impossible for the judge to consider Mr. Yost's circumstances to be tenable. A mentally ill person, it was argued, could never hold a job for long.

The assumption of mental illness also affects the way court personnel portray the adequacy of one's sources of other basic necessities. A source may be described as vulnerable if the patient's assumed mental illness might affect it. For example, court personnel argue that housing situations are untenable if they are easily disrupted by disturbed or erratic behavior. Thus, court personnel argue that persons who rent apartments on their own (even if they can document their ability to pay rent) should be committed, but persons who occupy institutional or structured settings may be described as relatively secure. Living in rental property, they say, requires financial responsibility and respect for formal and informal rules of apartment life. DAs and judges often argue that these mundane and minimal obligations are likely to pose major difficulties for mentally ill persons. They contend that patients will almost certainly disrupt the situation, thus jeopardizing their living arrangements and effectively depriving themselves of the adequate shelter required for their release. Presumptions regarding the needs of the mentally ill thus impose a compelling set of descriptive and evaluative constraints upon commitment arguments.

Other aspects of tenability considerations are similarly influenced. The adequacy of a caretaker, for example, is portrayed in terms of those capabilities required to deal with a potentially erratic, disruptive, violent person—even though no formal psychiatric prognosis suggests that such behavior is likely. Or a patient's pledge to adhere to a program of psychiatric care will be depicted as a worthless promise due to the person's impaired mental capacity. Robert Castillo's case illustrates several ways in which mental illness ascriptions permeate these aspects of tenability deliberations.

Mr. Castillo, a thirty-seven-year-old Chicano, was judged gravely disabled in Metropolitan Court after he repeatedly came to the attention of the police for "threatening and harassing" people in his neighborhood. The judge's account for his ruling suggested that Mr. Castillo's living situation was untenable because no competent caretaker was available to monitor his daily activities or ensure his continued outpatient treatment. While the judge indicated that Mr. Castillo's wife tried her best to keep track of him, he also noted that she was away from home at her job a good portion of the day. The judge said this was inadequate supervision, given her husband's mental condition:

[7:10]   [Metropolitan Court; J2, DA4, PD1, Dr7, Robert Castillo]

J2:

A guy like this may seem to be just fine one minute, then go off the deep end the next. If there's no one there watching all the time, who's gonna step in and take over when he loses his senses? Somebody has got to be constantly on guard.

The judge's assumption about Mr. Castillo's mental illness—both concerning its presence and the ways it affected Mr. Castillo—called for especially rigorous supervision in any living arrangement that was to be judged tenable. And it was the assumption, and not actual testimony, that supported the characterization of Mr. Castillo as gravely disabled.

That assumption also abetted the judge's challenge to Mr. Castillo's promise to get psychiatric care:

[7:11]   [Metropolitan Court; J2, DA4, PD1, Dr7, Robert Castillo]

J2:
> He needs treatment—regular medication—but he doesn't recognize that. In his mental state, he doesn't think he needs help. So he can't be trusted, and if she's [Mrs. Castillo] not around, who's gonna get him to the clinic? Who's gonna give him his meds? He says he'll take them now, but what about next week when he says he's better, when his delusions make him think that he feels OK and doesn't need them?

By inferring aspects of Mr. Castillo's psychiatric disturbance, and characterizing the symptoms of that disturbance in the fashion that he did, the judge displayed no hope for community treatment in the present circumstances. He argued that mental illness causes its victims to be oblivious to their own condition and needs, so one can never trust a person believed to be mentally ill to seek needed psychiatric help. And when one is assumed to be mentally ill, others (especially judges) are likely to interpret any report of a subjective sense of well-being, improvement, or remission as misapprehension, delusion, or irrationality—one further symptom of psychiatric disorder.

* * * * *

Despite the mental illness assumption and its interpretive implications, not all patients are committed. Even though mental illness ascriptions dictate stringent criteria for determining a living situation's tenability, a variety of arguments for release successfully portray appropriate situations for placing the "mentally ill" person in question. Chapter 8 examines some features of interpretive practice that are implicated in the descriptive construction of people and places that must be fit together in order to accomplish tenability.

Notes

1.   The contours of some of the assumptions have been discussed in Chapter 3.

2.   As Chapter 3 indicated, the mental illness assumption is accompanied by a general predisposition to try to help patients—to do something for them. A widespread concern for safeguarding the patients' "best interests" is closely associated with the assumption that they are mentally ill. Thus, the assumption is not perceived as intrinsically harmful to patients, and its use is seldom questioned.

Chapter 8

Constructing Tenability:
Interpretive Practice in Cultural Context

Orienting to the tenability of proposed living arrangements, commitment proceedings have a decidedly situational focus. Chapter 7, however, reasserted the importance of patients' mental condition, demonstrating how assumptions about mentally ill persons are consequential interpretive frameworks. This chapter describes how the orientation to tenability results in the simultaneous interpretation of both personal and situational factors within the broader context of commonsense knowledge about the social and cultural circumstances in which involuntary commitment is proposed. Tenability cannot be construed as merely a constructed feature of a physical environment. Rather, it is a practical conflation of personal and situational factors into a holistic representation of an adequate match between person and place. In these terms, tenability is constituted by formulating a plausible correspondence between a particular person—as he or she may be portrayed in court—and a living situation and its occupants' described ability to accommodate that person.

Hearing participants must describe patients in close conjunction with their arguments about living arrangements. Patients are typified in terms of characteristics like age, gender, and cultural background, which are argued to be related to their specific needs. The environment must then be portrayed as capable of accommodating a culturally recognized type of person—who is more than simply a mentally ill person—if hospitalization is to be ruled out.

As Chapter 6 noted, the decision-making process superficially resembles a search for and contingent discovery of a match between person and living situation. As the current chapter will demonstrate, however, the match or mismatch that is "turned up" is more of a descriptive, rhetorical accomplishment than it is a discovery. Court personnel argue

149

for and against commitment by strategically articulating patients' attributes with the accommodations they depict, any "fit" between the two being a product of interpretive practice.

Portraying patients, their significant others, and the living circumstances they propose to occupy is both artful (Garfinkel 1967) and rhetorical (Burke 1950; Miller 1991). Descriptions must make sense; they are accountable in that they must convince socially defined competent observers that the circumstances in question warrant the attributions and categorizations attached to them. Discourse and actual interpretable occurrences are thus mutually constraining and elaborating (Bilmes 1986). Persons and situations take on their known character as they are descriptively constituted, while, simultaneously, description and categorization orient to "what everyone knows" about the types of people and circumstances in question if descriptions are to be compelling. The acceptability or accountability of descriptions derives—at least in part—from the way they align with culturally shared vocabularies and understandings of people, situations, and issues whose relevance to commitment proceedings can be demonstrated.

Commitment hearings take place within a contemporary American cultural milieu. As participants articulate their concerns and describe the parties and circumstances of the case at hand, they invoke the conventional, normal, and commonplace—cultural hallmarks like gender, age, home, and family, for example—as standards against which persons, behaviors, and circumstances can be compared. This chapter examines how culturally normal forms are utilized as interpretive resources, turning first to "person description" as a cornerstone of the commitment decision-making process, then examining the descriptive construction of "community-based accommodations" as complementary components of tenability assessments.

Producing People

"People processing" (Hasenfeld 1972) in organizational settings is often analyzed in terms of how organization members deal with persons who receive the organization's services, whether they are generally desired services such as those provided by welfare or health care agencies, or the undesired attention of social control agents like the police, courts, or commitment hearings. The analyses presume that persons come or are brought to these organizations with identifiable—though often problematic—characteristics, problems, and/or complaints. Street-level bureaucrats (Lipsky 1980)—social workers, therapists, social control personnel, and the like—then decipher and discern the nature of the troubles and what can be done about them. In this sort of analysis, street-level bureaucrats' work largely consists of articulating the "facts" of cases with appropriate organizational policies (Lipsky 1980). The work is framed as a kind of sorting process whereby the "actual" circumstances, causes, and consequences of everyday human difficulties are systematically and professionally revealed so that organizationally appropriate responses may be prescribed.

This perspective treats the practical worlds of organizational workers as a constellation of persons, circumstances, and actions that exist independently of workers' concern for them. Alternatively, people processing work can be analyzed as work involving interpretive practice that produces the situationally relevant characteristics and circumstances of persons for the practical purposes at hand. From this viewpoint, persons' distinctive and organizationally relevant features are descriptively accomplished in situ in the course of processing cases. In some instances, this amounts to the rhetorical production of organizational clients and their problems, as well as candidate solutions for these troubles (Loseke 1989, 1992; Miller 1991). In this sense, organizational actors are as much people *producers* as people processors (Holstein 1992).

Person-Description

Involuntary commitment proceedings are prototypic instances of people processing. Various human service professionals—social workers, psychiatric personnel, attorneys, judges, police, and others—attend to, evaluate, and suggest organizational responses to the persons who might be committed. If commitment hearings eventuate, court personnel repeatedly and routinely describe the persons with whom they are concerned. These person-descriptions (Maynard 1984) provide the justification for organizational actions. For the practical purpose at hand, interpretive practice assembles the reality (or at least aspects of it) that warrants commitment arguments.

Person-descriptions may be offered as objective or dispassionate reports of the "facts" of the case at hand; many descriptions pass virtually unnoticed, matter-of-fact statements that attract the attention of neither speaker nor hearers. Alternatively, they may be explicitly incorporated into partisan commitment arguments. In either case, they provide situated points of view rather than disembodied, objective arrays of the "facts" of the case at hand. Any description may thus be considered rhetorical, as it advocates a particular version of the persons, experience, or circumstances in question. Description must therefore be analyzed as purposeful action.

Person-descriptions tend to be formulated economically (Sacks and Schegloff 1979), often through the use of a limited number of well-known categories or typifications. The use of a particular category implies a constellation of ancillary features that are typically associated with the category (e.g., "elderly lady" might imply harmlessness). The application of a categorical description thus provides a basis for ascribing other characteristics, activities, and motives to persons (Sacks 1972).

Person-descriptions are not assembled indiscriminately, nor are they bounded by standards of descriptive adequacy (Atkinson and Drew 1979). Rather they are occasioned by the task at hand, and produced to address immediately relevant issues. To paraphrase Maynard (1984, p. 138), who a person is, for the purpose of organizational processing, depends upon what the organization is trying to accomplish. What a patient is, for the practical purposes of commitment hearings, is therefore *argued*, not merely presented.

Organizational Perspective

Mary Douglas (1986) suggests that one's social location provides distinctive ways of interpreting and talking about practically relevant matters—an institutional discourse or "gaze" (Foucault 1973) embodied by the organized features of one's social circumstances. While participants in commitment hearings encounter a common set of organizational constraints, they also import diverse agendas and distinctive organizational and professional backgrounds. Thus, they articulate their concerns in ways that reflect contrasting perspectives and goals.

Depictions of the significant features of commitment cases consequently vary according to the contextual contingencies of their production. Tenability, for example, is not a singular construct, but instead comprises a combination of related concerns that may be articulated differently by the various hearing participants. Among the most prominent of these concerns are patients' *manageability, vulnerability,* and *remedial prospects* (Holstein 1987a, 1988b), and living situations' ability to accommodate these characteristics. Participants may find the concerns differentially compelling, so person-descriptions are not constructed or implicated in an automatic or fixed fashion. Advancing age may be used to characterize one patient's vulnerability, but a similar description— "going on sixty," for example—may be used to characterize another as easily managed, a quality arguably expected from a man that old.

Judges, in general, say they are primarily concerned with controlling the trouble that accompanies psychiatric disturbance, so they tend to mention aspects of a case that are particularly germane to managing such trouble. Psychiatrists, on the other hand, are more therapeutically oriented, and may be more likely to argue about patients' remedial prospects. Contrasting concerns may translate into diverging discourses of tenability, with one party using a vocabulary of treatment, prognosis, and remission, while the other speaks of custody and care.

Some hearing participants are likely to articulate the vulnerability of mentally ill persons with reference to a particular set of traits, while others may invoke the same characteristics in arguments relating to manageability, and so forth. A DA, for example may imply that a female patient is especially vulnerable—as women are typically said to be—and thus needs to be hospitalized. Conversely, a PD may take the same descriptive category and use it to establish the expectation of manageability, suggesting that women are usually easy to take care of. Organizational and professional perspectives, then, suggest distinctive ways for commitment participants to argue cases.

Using Normal Forms

Commitment proceedings rely upon global characterizations of types of people, typifications (Schutz 1970) rhetorically constructed to address the practical issues at hand. Whether cast as "a guy who seems to have gotten it together" or "the kind of person that will end up back in the hospital," for example, patients are described in terms that apply to social types, not as lists of traits and characteristics. These descriptions rely upon typical understandings of the normal constituents of members of categories to convey intended meanings, interpreting the person sought to be committed by relating him or her to culturally known "normal forms."

Consider the case of Polly Brown (see Appendix 1), who was charged with grave disability because of her bizarre, agitated behavior and her inability to get along with others. Part of the argument to commit included the accusation that Ms. Brown had threatened staff members on the psychiatric ward where she had spent the past few days. Ms. Brown's PD attempted to argue that her outburst was understandable in light of its context, the behavior one might expect from a "normal" person under the circumstances:

[8:1]   [Metropolitan Court; J1, DA4, PD2, Dr16, Polly Brown]

PD2:
> As for her [Ms. Brown's] behavior in the hospital, we have heard that a nurse called her children bastards. I believe anyone would be agitated if they heard this sort of talk. She's protective like any mother would be. Any woman with children would be upset.

The PD's argument both displayed the situational contingencies that made Ms. Brown's alleged outburst understandable and presented the reaction as that of a normal person in that particular situation; anyone (especially any mother) would do the same thing, or so he claimed.

Besides references to normal persons or typical actions, standard categories—gender, age, and group membership, for example—are frequently used to interpret and assess patients and their prospects for commitment (Holstein 1987a, 1990a). Either explicitly, or by tacit implication, culturally assumed notions about the normal or conventional behaviors and traits of persons of a particular class or group are used to establish standards against which patients are evaluated. In Polly Brown's case, the categorization devices (Sacks 1972) *mother* and *family* were used to interpret the reasonableness of the patient's actions (she was being "protective," an expectable reaction from a "mother" when her "children" were disparaged). Alternatively, severe troubles are made visible by noting departures from the expected (e.g., "People who can take care of themselves don't say and do the kind of things he does"). Using contrasts and comparisons, participants assemble descriptions that depict persons and their circumstances, providing implicit instructions for how to understand what is being described.

Everyday Categories as Interpretive Resources: Gender and Age

Both explicit reference to normal types and the tacit use of standard categories serve to contextualize interpretations of persons and behaviors. Indeed, even the seemingly most casual acts of classification provide interpretive resources for understanding and arguing commitment issues. Patients are always classified according to sex, for example, even if this is done unwittingly or as an act of ostensibly simple description. Gender is invariably noted in simple forms of address (e.g., Ms. Smith, Mr. Jones) or repeated use of personal pronouns (e.g., "He has a long history," "She has four children"). Gender references are so routine and commonplace that they go virtually unnoticed, constituting "factual" representations that attract no special attention and appear on the surface to be unimportant. Yet both tacitly and explicitly, gender depictions serve as significant interpretive resources that organize perceptions and understandings of patients' traits, symptoms, biographies, and behaviors in distinctive and meaningful ways.

As a scheme of interpretation, gender provides a way of understanding features of the person to whom it has been assigned. In the commitment process, it may contextualize particular traits, symptoms, and behaviors, providing an interpretive frame of reference for how they should be construed. Arguments concerning psychiatric diagnosis or a patient's ability to live successfully in a community setting, for example, often proceed explicitly within the framework of gender depictions. Quite simply, what may be considered mentally healthy *for a man* might be diagnosed as pathological *for a woman*, and vice versa. A living situation that might be considered viable for a psychiatrically troubled man may be portrayed as untenable for a mentally ill woman, and so on.

Consider, for example, a case involving Gerald Simms. The testifying psychiatrist initially characterized Simms as a "severely troubled man" and gave the following account of his diagnosis of schizophrenia:

[8:2] [Metropolitan Court; J2, DA1, PD5, Dr11, Gerald Simms]

Dr11:

> Mr. Simms suffers from drastic mood swings. His affect is extremely labile. One minute he'll be in tears, the next he's just fine. He fluctuates. His affect may be flattened, then elevated. One moment he'll be telling you about his cleaning business, then he'll flip out of character and cry like a brokenhearted schoolgirl over the most insignificant thing. Something that should never upset a grown man like Mr. Simms. During his periods of flattened affect, he seems to lose all interest. . . . His passivity—he's almost docile in a very sweet sort of way. He just smiles and lets everything pass. It's completely inappropriate for an adult male.

While the relevance of Mr. Simms's gender to the psychiatrist's diagnosis was not immediately apparent, it subsequently became clear that the diagnosis was assembled by articulating gender with specific interpretations of conduct that made sense of Mr. Simms's behaviors in light of the "type" of person (i.e., a gendered person) involved.

A patient's age may also be cited to establish the sense in which particular behaviors can be seen as symptoms of specific mental illnesses (Holstein 1990a). Testifying psychiatrists, for example, use age or life course location (like they use gender) to display a patient's behavior as "inappropriate" and hence psychologically unhealthy. For example, a Dr. Haas employed this practice in the following testimony:

[8:3] [Metropolitan Court; J2, DA1, PD7, Dr13, Jake Donner]

Dr13:

> Jake has the, shall we say, the enthusiasm of a much younger man. His landlord says he's out every night, and sometimes doesn't come back until the next morning. When I examined Mr. Donner he made no secret of his, let's say, passion for members of the opposite sex. He was extremely distraught about being hospitalized because he said he was dating several women and they would all be upset if he stopped coming round to visit them. He said some pretty outrageous things for a man his age. He

claimed that he needed to have sex at least once a day or he would, as he put it, lose his manhood. And he said these women were anxious to oblige him. Now, here's a man in his fifties—what is he, fifty five, sixty—saying the kind of things you'd expect from some teenager bragging to his buddies, but I'd have to say they were clearly inappropriate from him.

Dr. Haas went on to say Mr. Donner was mentally ill and gravely disabled, substantiating his assessment by citing, among other things, Mr. Donner's inappropriate sexual desires and delusions.

Throughout his testimony, the psychiatrist elucidated much of Mr. Donner's symptomatology with reference to age. He established its diagnostic relevance by articulating a connection between Mr. Donner's age and interpretations of his affect and behavior. Dr. Haas argued, for example, that Mr. Donner's tales of his sexual exploits were "outrageous" for a "man his age." Age implicitly underpinned his standards of appropriateness. The sexual talk was not intrinsically outrageous, but was portrayed as such only when it was linked to expectations for an older person who presumably was not erotically inclined. Age thus provided an interpretive benchmark for understanding the conduct and claims in question.

Categorization devices like age and gender provide commonsense models for depicting what culturally known types of people are like, and how members of such categories may be expected to behave. Participants in commitment hearings consult these models and argue how the case at hand is consistent with or departs from what would generally be considered typical or normal.

Contrast Structures

While patients are often compared favorably to normal types, participants in commitment hearings, especially DAs and psychiatrists, are more likely to use these models as standards for negative comparison. Personal and interpersonal deficiencies can be descriptively accomplished, in part, by pointing out how a patient's traits or behaviors are anomalous—that is, unmotivated by the circumstances as described. Hearing participants routinely employ rhetorical devices that Dorothy Smith (1978) calls *contrast structures* to achieve this end.

Contrast structures juxtapose characterizations of traits or behavior with statements that supply instructions for seeing the traits or behavior as anomalous or problematic (Smith 1978). Normal forms, typifications, or "standard pattern rules" are expectations held in advance about what events or behaviors follow from the expected model. Anomalies—or in the case of commitment proceedings, instances of incompetence or inappropriateness—are accomplished by constructing relationships between rules or definitions of situations and descriptions of an individual's behavior so that the former do not properly provide for the latter. It is "evident," then, that the behavior is anomalous.

The contrastive device operates in the preceding section of this chapter, where notions of typical gender- and age-related factors were used to accentuate the problems of those being described. In extract [8:2], the psychiatrist explicitly contrasted descriptions of Mr. Simms's behavior with normal expectations for a person of his gender and age. Mr. Simms's emotions, for example, were portrayed as those of "a broken-hearted schoolgirl" crying over matters that should "never upset a grown man." His "passivity" was "inappropriate for an adult male." Mr. Simms's gender was made salient and consequential to the diagnosis as it was displayed, juxtaposed and contrasted with descriptions of behavior as female-like or not properly masculine. Apparent incongruities were then cited as documents of mental illness.

Normative gender standards were used to organize the understanding of Mr. Simms and his behavior, instructing hearers to note the ways in which he acted "inappropriately." Gender was an implicit interpretive framework, imparting distinctive meanings to particular behaviors and indexing those behaviors as symptoms of mental illness for "a person of this type" or indications of mental health for "a person of that gender." Frequently, in commitment proceedings, what was considered sane or normal for a man might be described as unhealthy for a woman, and vice versa.

Age is similarly used, normative expectations for persons of specified ages highlighting incongruities in patients' behavior, affect, or demeanor. In extract [8:3], Jake Donner's age and conduct were juxtaposed and compared with descriptions of behavior considered normal or appropriate for someone of a *different* age group. Apparent similarities—where contrasts were expected—were noted as signs of Mr. Donner's inappropriate behavior, and were ultimately cited as symptoms of his illness. Mr. Donner's "enthusiasm" (I took this to mean his sexual proclivities), for example, was portrayed as that of a "much younger man." In the ensuing discussion, Dr. Haas used this to document Mr. Donner's mental disturbance, framing it as age inappropriate and symptomatic of psychiatric distress. In addition, Dr. Haas compared Mr. Donner's claims about sexual needs and prowess to those of a boastful adolescent. The contrast drawn between what was considered normal for "a man in his fifties" and a "teenager" underscored the disturbed character of Mr. Donner's claim. While the age appropriateness of Mr. Donner's behavior was not the sole concern in this case, Dr. Haas clearly made age salient to his evaluation of Mr. Donner's mental status; his testimony *produced* the relevance of Jake Donner's age, using normative expectations to establish the unsuitability of Mr. Donner's reported behavior.

When age is made relevant, commitment proceedings are often concerned with whether a person is "on or off course" (Gubrium and Holstein 1993) in terms of the typical or expected aging cycle. Psychiatrists regularly portray patients going off course to substantiate their diagnoses. For example, in another Metropolitan Court case, Dr. Peters diagnosed William Frederic, forty-nine years old, as schizophrenic, citing, among other reasons, her belief that Mr. Frederic was "acting progressively more immature" and "not acting his age." According to the psychiatrist, Mr. Frederic caused a public disturbance by "childishly" refusing to ride as a passenger in his own car while his daughter drove the vehicle. He refused to sit quietly in the passenger's seat, and tried to wrestle the steering wheel away from his daughter as she drove the car out of the driveway. He clung to the steering wheel, which sounded the car's horn, and refused to budge as the car came to rest in the middle of the street. His outburst became so vociferous that traffic backed up, a crowd of neighbors gathered, and someone called the police.

Dr. Peters argued that while Mr. Frederic's insistence on driving himself might be understandable, his highly agitated, animated outburst and his refusal to come out from behind the steering wheel violated standards of decorum and judgment expected from "someone his age." Note that the doctor might have characterized the behavior as disturbed in its own right—that is, without explicitly invoking a particular interpretive context—yet she chose to underscore its inappropriateness by contrasting it with age-related expectations. Dr. Peters suggested, both explicitly and tacitly, that as people grow older, they normally develop "mature" responses to frustration that do not involve uncontrollable public outbursts. Mr. Frederic, she implied, was veering off course by becoming progressively more "immature," a clear sign of disabling mental disorder.

Normal Forms and Tenability Assessments

References to normal forms insinuate tenability discussions as well as psychiatric assessments. Again, gender and age—among other standards—provide normative expectations for what constitutes a viable community living option. For example, involuntary commitment was proposed for Kathleen Wells, a thirty-two-year-old white female, when she was found living in a large cardboard carton beneath a railroad overpass. While she was diagnosed as severely mentally ill and several problems were noted, her hearing in Northern Court eventually focused on the viability of the shelter. Arguing for commitment, the DA indicated several structural and sanitary deficiencies in the proposed dwelling, then used the patient's gender as a framework for claiming this arrangement as especially untenable.

[8:4]   [Northern Court; J1, DA1, PD2, Dr2, Kathleen Wells]

DA1:

Now I know Miss Wells claims that this [the cardboard box] is as good as the subsidized public housing programs the DSS [Department of Social Services] has suggested she look into, but we have to consider more than its construction aspects. . . . You can't allow a woman to be exposed to all the other things that go on out there under the [railroad] tracks. Many of those men have lived like that for years, but we're talking about a woman here. A sick and confused woman who doesn't realize the trouble she's asking for. She simply cannot live like that. That's no place for a woman, especially after dark. . . . She's not taking it [being a woman in the midst of men] into account. She doesn't realize how dangerous it is for her. It's up to the court to protect her.

The argument here was that the proposed living arrangement, while perhaps being tolerable for men, was inappropriate *for a woman*. Indeed, the dangerous character of the setting—and its consequent untenability—was not fully apparent until the setting was described as the potential residence of a *woman*. The DA had to invoke gender to clearly establish the unsuitability of the situation. The tenability of the setting per se was not being evaluated, for it could not be meaningfully removed from the context of its occupant's gender.

Age is similarly used in tenability arguments. Martin Evans, for instance, had apparently lived uneventfully for several years in a small apartment, regularly taking medications that a VA hospital psychiatrist had prescribed for him. His commitment was sought after a series of disturbances at a local community recreation center. The troubles climaxed when Mr. Evans refused to leave the facility at closing time, saying he was the owner and could spend the night if he wanted. The police took Mr. Evans to his apartment, but when they entered, they discovered that the electricity and telephone had been disconnected, and there was nothing to eat in the apartment. At the commitment hearing, the DA sought Mr. Evans's hospitalization on the grounds that "a man in Mr. Evans's condition" was gravely disabled; he wasn't able to live unsupervised in the community. Age was invoked to display the inadequacy of the situation:

[8:5]   [Metropolitan Court; J2, DA3, PD1, Dr19, Martin Evans]

DA3:

> There's just no way the man can take care of himself right now. Look what
> happened. He just let everything go. Your honor, the man's getting up in
> years and that place [the apartment] will simply not suffice. He doesn't
> eat. He doesn't pay his bills. It's a wonder the old guy didn't get himself in
> worse shape than he already is. It might not seem like much, him being a
> pain in the neck at the rec center, but the fact is, with a man his age we can
> probably expect this sort of thing to continue if nothing's done about it.
> And if he goes back to that apartment, nothing's gonna change. In three
> months the lights will be off and he'll be back on the streets.

Here, the DA purposefully described the apartment in terms of its
inability to meet the needs of a man "getting up in years," strongly
implying that the living situation contributed to Mr. Evans's recent disturbances and openly predicting that troubles would recur if Mr. Evans
returned to the apartment. First invoking age as a relevant person-
description, the DA then claimed that the situation was inappropriate
for "a man his age." The assessment of living circumstances was thoroughly linked to the kind of person to be accommodated. In this case,
the normal expectations for a person of Mr. Evans's age provided the
interpretive framework for arguing that the apartment in question was a
place that "will simply not suffice."

Of course normal standards may also be invoked to patients' advantage. Commitment was recommended in the two cases discussed immediately above because the patients' living situations were portrayed as
inappropriate for particular types (i.e., gender and age, respectively) of
persons. But normative models can be used just as convincingly to demonstrate the viability of living arrangements. For example, a Metropolitan Court judge released Sharlene Fox, a twenty-seven-year-old
black female, justifying his decision by noting that she would be able to
live with her mother and aunt:

[8:6]   [Metropolitan Court; J1, DA1, PD4, Dr8, Sharlene Fox]

J1:

> I'm releasing this woman if she'll go and stay with her family, her mother
> and her aunt. They'll take her in . . . and give her a good place to stay. But
> you gotta do what they say [to Ms. Fox], or you'll be right back in here.
> Her mother should be able to deal with her this time. Her [Sharlene's]
> husband's not around [he had been portrayed as an irresponsible trouble-
> maker] and she should be able to take care of her daughter all right. Her
> symptoms seem to be under control and I think that between the two of
> them they can manage her. It's not like she's some two-hundred-pound
> guy who they'd have to put in a straitjacket if he got off his medica-

tion. . . . We're talking about a woman here who isn't going to be able to cause much trouble.

Ms. Fox's gender was invoked here to describe her as easily managed—a culturally expected pattern and an important feature of the proposal that she live with her mother and aunt. The judge used gender to argue that a woman, unlike a man, might be appropriately housed in this situation. Comparison to the normal type was used to forestall commitment.

Person-descriptions and references to normal forms appear to be constrained primarily by speakers' pragmatic interests. Recall that Kathleen Wells was portrayed as vulnerable because she was a woman, while Sharlene Fox's manageability was seen as part of being female. Altogether different meanings of female were accomplished, both of them within culturally accepted understandings of "what everyone knows" about women. Clearly gender, like other descriptive categories, is multidimensional, its specific aspects emerging only upon the occasions of its use.

More generally, the meaning of all personal characteristics is essentially indeterminate. Rather than being "cultural dopes" (Garfinkel 1967) responding automatically in terms of culturally promoted images, hearing participants exercise vast creative discretion in how they assign and depict personal attributes, and in how they bring particular depictions to bear upon the case at hand.[1]

Accomplishing Accommodations: Matching People with Places

Tenability, as a practical conflation of personal and situational factors, is constituted by formulating an appropriate *match* between a particular patient—as he or she may be portrayed in court—and a living situation's described ability to accommodate that person. Consequently, the parameters of proposed living situations are a focal point of most commitment proceedings. To establish the viability of a living situation, participants must argue, at least in part, that the arrangement accommodates the patient's special needs. Recall, for example, that in extract [8:5], the DA argued that Martin Evans's apartment living situation was ill-suited to deal with Mr. Evans's special needs, predicting that further troubles would ensue if Mr. Evans was allowed to return to that setting. The essence of the argument was that the living situation was untenable because it could not adequately accommodate a man of Mr. Evans's age and special problems. Conversely, in a similar case involving sixty-year-old Calvin Howe, Mr. Howe's home was portrayed as a viable alternative to hospitalization because he was "a grown man, fully capable of taking care of himself." The PD portrayed the house as suitable for "kindly old Calvin," an easily managed man "going on sixty" who posed little threat of further disturbance. The house was described as a perfect match for Mr. Howe's special demands.

Tenability, then, is descriptively accomplished, depending upon the rhetorical depiction of both the setting and the demands to which it must respond. Like person-descriptions, depictions of living situations reflect practical commitment concerns; they are occasioned productions rather than literal representations. The rhetoric of commitment proceedings thus orients to the alignment of needs and accommodations with interpretive practice providing the "fit" or "disjuncture" between the two.

Tenability arguments interweave a distinctive constellation of concerns, relating and crosscutting issues regarding patients' basic necessities, caretakers, and ongoing treatment programs, linking specific issues to more general orientations. As they are described and considered, living arrangements (and their incumbents) are assessed, with varying emphases, for their custodial adequacy, permanence or durability, and capacity for genuine compassion and caring. Various participants in commitment proceedings are likely to ask and/or respond to the following questions:

- How, and how well, is a proposed living situation, and those in it, going to "look out" for the patient?
- Will someone be there to "keep an eye on him (or her)" to head off potentially serious troubles?
- How long can a particular arrangement be counted on?
- Will the patient be treated with true "caring" or will he or she become a bother—just "get in the way"?

These concerns are central to the rhetorical moves employed in arguments over the tenability of proposed living arrangements.

Home and Family: Hallmarks of Deinstitutionalized Care

With the issue of community placement dominating commitment proceedings, participants compare and contrast various deinstitutionalized living options with hospitalization. While independent living situations, nursing homes, board and care facilities, and other sheltered living arrangements are routinely considered, commitment proceedings almost invariably explore the possibility of placing the patient at "home" in the care of his or her "family." Home and family—as hallmarks of caring and concern—are used as standards against all other options can be compared. The discourse of home care thus serves as a resource for articulating tenability-related issues, implicating images of family and household in the commitment process (Holstein 1990b).

Participants routinely mobilize images of home and family as they explore matches between patients and proposed living arrangements. While these represent only a limited range of possible alternatives, and nothing mandates the consideration of home care, its possibility is repeatedly made relevant. Participants frequently argue about whether a patient's home and family can provide him or her with basic needs, caretakers, and assistance with treatment regimens, suggesting, at least obliquely, a set of cultural assumptions about the relation between individuals, families, and households.[2] Facets of home and family are thus used to express culturally shared notions about concerned care. Just as shared assumptions about types of persons are used to discern and specify patients' characteristics, problems, and needs, images of congenial environments are invoked to interpret available placement options.

Care in the patient's family home, for example, is routinely—and often passionately—argued to be the best, most healthful of all possible living situations. Consider how this was done by the PD representing Leon Mason, as he articulated the possibilities for home care against the special problems and demands that Mason presented:

[8:7]   [Metropolitan Court, J1, DA7, PD5, Dr14, Leon Mason]

PD5:

> We're proposing that Mr. Mason go home and work out his problems in surroundings that are more conducive to some kind of recovery. . . . Getting him back home has a lot to offer. First, it's clear that his family wants him home. His wife and kids miss him, and he misses them. That alone gives him a sense of security and reduces his anxiety level and it seems that he's most likely to have problems when he gets anxious. There's something to be said for home cooking and sleeping in your own bed. . . . People at home love him, care about him. That's got to count for something. They're his family, they love him, care about him. We know Mr. Mason has gotten out of control in the past, but with his sister living at home now, there'll be someone there to watch out for him all the time, someone always around who he knows, cares about him. . . . I think we can even expect Mr. Mason to be more cooperative if he's at home. He says he just feels more comfortable there. . . . He says he'll take his meds if his wife reminds him. . . . He's more likely to follow through and not go off the program again.

This description of life at home not only enumerated its advantages over the mental hospital, but also spoke directly to the court's tenability concerns. The PD argued that placement at home with his family ensured Mason's basic needs and supervision, representing a sort of home-based therapeutic regimen, complete with medication plan and affectional treatment. But more than this, the repeated use of home and family imagery underscored the depth of commitment present, and the security to be imparted. "Home cooking," for example, implied more than adequate nutrition, conveying a sense of love and personal attention. Having "family" around meant that concern and care would be real and enduring, not fleeting or insubstantial.

References to home and family also supply the background against which the accommodative inadequacies of a community placement are displayed. This is evident in the following explanation offered by a Metropolitan Court judge for his decision to commit Victor Ruiz:

[8:8]   [Metropolitan Court; J2, DA2, PD2, Dr15, Victor Ruiz]

J2:

> I'm very skeptical about this plan to move across town to take an apartment. Do we know anything more about this roommate? It really doesn't matter. I'd be more comfortable if we were talking about familiar surroundings, some kind of home life, [directed at Ruiz:]but what you're proposing is to start from scratch and I'm not sure you're up to it. . . . If I was sending you home it might be different, but they won't have you and as well-meaning as your friend may be, these things usually don't work out. At home you'd have someone to take care of you, someone who'd be there for the duration. I don't feel like we can count on that right now.

Here, the home was explicitly offered as a standard against which Mr. Ruiz's living situation was compared. Criteria for establishing tenability were implicitly argued in terms of the home; the proposed living arrangement was then compared, this time unfavorably, thus providing substantial warrant for a decision to commit.

Family rhetoric was also used in this fashion. Dr. Raj, for instance, invoked "lack of family" to argue that Paula Jones should be committed:

[8:9]   [Metropolitan Court; J1, DA1, PD3, Dr20, Paula Jones]

Dr20:

> Paula can barely function on the ward. If she is released she will have no one to look after her. Her family, she has no family. They are all in New Orleans except for her sister who she was living with. But she is going back because she doesn't want to have anything more to do with her. She has no one to look out for her.

Once again, family was invoked as a standard of concerned care. Its absence signaled a deficiency in Ms. Jones's living situation that, according to the doctor, could not be ignored.

The rhetorics of home and family are thus used to attach particular significance to settings and social relations within them. In the course of commitment proceedings, participants routinely describe a variety of circumstances as familial or homelike, conferring distinctive meaning upon settings as different as private residences, board and care facilities, and even mental hospitals. Interpretively transformed, the descriptively "domesticated" circumstances are then related to the commitment issues at hand. Consider, for example, the interpretive transformation accomplished by the PD in the following description of the board and care facility that was proposed as the future residence of patient John Becker:

[8:10]   [Metropolitan Court; J2, DA3, PD1, Dr7, John Becker]

PD1:
> Valley View has agreed that John can return once he's back on his medication program. This is the perfect place for him. They know him there, they take good care of him, and he wants to go back. It's been like home to him, certainly more of a home than he had living with his parents. . . . The staff there have become his family.

By casting the board and care facility as Mr. Becker's "home"—indeed more of a home than the house in which he was raised—the PD secured a range of understandings about the quality of life, especially its affective and therapeutic aspects, that Becker would experience at Valley View. Calling the facility a home was more than a mere exchange of labels; it fundamentally transformed the meaning of the place. Labeling the staff "his family" effected a similar reformulation. Calling dwellings "homes" and their inhabitants "families" (or denying such depictions) insinuates a set of meanings and potentials that speak poignantly to caregiving and tenability concerns.

While participants in commitment proceedings regularly portray the material advantages of living at home or with family, they are apt to use home and family discourse to address a constellation of less tangible aspects of the mental health care experience as well. To speak of care provided "at home" typically suggests more than simply the availability of adequate lodging. The image is more encompassing, suggesting that one will be afforded a comprehensive range of material, therapeutic, and emotional necessities and comforts. Both home and family may be anthropomorphized at times, giving each abilities and capacities associated with volitional, personal caregiving and conveying the compassionate, affectional, nurturant character of enduring familial relations (Gubrium and Holstein 1990). Home and family are thus used to denote "real" caring, not merely instrumental custodianship.

But such meanings do not automatically attach to all instances where home or family are invoked. Home and family might also be associated with patients' emotional security, autonomy, self-control, or dignity, for example. As exemplars of reliable, salutary accommodations, or as standards for violation, home and family offer a variety of rhetorically useful images for justifying commitment decisions. But because the images are formulated in response to particular situations and circumstances, they resist general typologies or categorization. The meaning of home or family for the purposes of commitment proceedings is realized only through their actual articulation with the case at hand. How they are descriptively employed, then, is essentially indeterminate, depending upon how diverse understandings of home or family are formulated and applied.

Home and Family as Rhetoric

Depictions of home and family are not merely descriptive or expository. Rather, domestic order is produced, transformed, and sustained for decidedly practical purposes; home and family are used to organize, influence, and *advocate* interpretations and decisions. Tom Cline's commitment hearing illustrates the extent to which they are rhetorical resources. Dr. Brown testified in Metropolitan Court that Mr. Cline, a twenty-seven-year-old white male, was gravely disabled, noting that he was chronically schizophrenic and was alternately in states of agitation, delusion, and disorientation. Dr. Brown argued that Mr. Cline's physical and mental well-being would be jeopardized if he were not given close institutional supervision. Near the end of Dr. Brown's testimony, the judge asked if there was anyone who might take care of Mr. Cline if he were released. Dr. Brown replied:

[8:11]   [Metropolitan Court; J1, DA1, PD5, Dr8, Tom Cline]

Dr8:
    Not to my knowledge. He has no one, no family to speak of. He might try
    to move in with his mother but she hasn't been willing to participate in his
    treatment up to this point.

Dr. Brown used family somewhat ironically to argue that Mr. Cline could not possibly live with his mother. Although she might be kin, casting the mother as "no family" clearly implied that she had not provided adequate support in the past and therefore could not be expected to act like family—that is, gratuitously support and cooperate with a treatment regimen—in the future. The meaning of family was implicitly linked to the custodial and therapeutic concerns that characterized Dr.

Brown's organizational and professional orientations. Describing Mr. Cline's situation as "no family" emphasized how untenable Mr. Cline's proposed living situation would be, rhetorically underscoring the need for hospitalization.

The judge was not satisfied with this assessment, however, and continued his questioning:

[8:12] [Metropolitan Court; J1, DA1, PD5, Dr8, Tom Cline]

J1:   Now let me get this straight. You say he wants to live with his mother?

Dr8: He's mentioned that on several occasions. But that's just not going to work. She hasn't gotten involved with any of his outpatient treatment plans in the past and she really doesn't seem interested. She may take him, but it won't last.

J1:   But she's willing to take care of him, let him live there [at her house], so he does have some family to turn to if we release him, right?

Dr8: Not really. His mother just doesn't care what we do for him. She's not going to help much.

J1:   What I'm trying to get at here is has she agreed that he can live there?

Dr8: Grudgingly. It's not going to be much of a home for this man.

Despite the judge's apparent skepticism, Dr. Brown maintained his depiction of Mr. Cline's mother as "no family to speak of," continuing to focus on therapeutic issues. The judge, however, revealed a different orientation to both the case at hand and, consequently, to family characterizations. His relative lack of concern for therapeutic matters permitted a different picture of Mr. Cline's mother, leaving open the possibility for arguing that Mr. Cline might be released to live in a community setting because he had "some family to turn to." Dr. Brown countered by noting that while Mr. Cline could live with his mother, it would not be "much of a home," again stripping the household of any implied concern or nurturance.

In this exchange, different aspects of the household were said to signal family according to the diverse interests of the participants. The judge, with his custodial orientation, noted family in the presence of a caretaker (that is, the mother), while the psychiatrist, with his therapeutic agenda, denied the existence of family even though he, too, acknowledged the mother's presence. In a sense, the judge and psychiatrist apprehended and argued the features of the scenario—the "facts" of the case—as disparate collections of experiential data, even though they addressed the same set of circumstances.

When he testified, Mr. Cline indicated his desire to live with his mother, who he claimed had agreed to take him in. Under cross-examination he asserted that he had never let his mother "boss him around" and that he did not want her "poking her nose into his business" and "nagging" him about his medications and doctor's appointments. In her summation, Mr. Cline's PD returned to images of home and family to argue that Mr. Cline had a viable living situation and should not be hospitalized:

[8:13]   [Metropolitan Court; J1, DA1, PD5, Dr8, Tom Cline]

PD5:
>So if he's released, Mr. Cline is going to be with family, back in his family home. . . . I think we have to consider how important it is that he'll be with family. He's got a kind of security there that you can't find anywhere else. Just being there is all it might take to get this man headed in the right direction.

The use of home and family was clearly rhetorical, a tactic adopted to convey the sense in which Mr. Cline's proposal for community living was especially appropriate. Discursively establishing a home and family for Mr. Cline simultaneously established the viability of his proposed living situation. To deny this would, in effect, challenge "what everyone knows" family to be.

The DA chose an alternative tactic in his summation. Instead of contesting family's implicit meanings, he challenged the legitimacy of the PD's family assignment:

[8:14]   [Metropolitan Court; J1, DA1, PD5, Dr8, Tom Cline]

DA1:
>If his mother lets him live there, it's not clear that she can do anything for him. It's one thing to say he has a family to look out for him, and another to say that his sixty-year-old mother is going to get him to stay on his program. She hasn't been all that attentive and he even admits that he doesn't want her bossing him around. . . . There's no way she can handle a guy like him if he gets upset. If someone else was around, family or somebody that could keep him under control, but not just her. . . . We'd all like to see Mr. Cline make it on the outside, but I'm afraid this is not the kind of family setting you'd want for him. Where is this family?

Here, the DA all but denied that a supportive family existed. Characterizing family in terms of care, control, and supervision of Mr. Cline's treatment program, he argued that there was no one available to provide these things, implying in the process that there was no real family present. By challenging the PD's argument regarding the very existence of family, he asserted that Mr. Cline's community living situation was untenable, without challenging the contention that a family environment would be a good one for Mr. Cline.

This exchange illustrates how rhetorically useful descriptions and images were superimposed on the same real-world referent to warrant claims and counterclaims regarding what the situation was really like. When family status was assigned to her, Mr. Cline's mother could be claimed as a placement resource—someone the court could call upon to help enact a form of community custody. Successfully challenging the assignment of home and family, however, could effectively deprive the court of this resource; tenability could not be established where "no family" existed. Ultimately, the "reality" of this case—and thus the "reality" of Mr. Cline's home and family—were practical, rhetorical accomplishments.

Description, Rhetoric, and Argumentation

Interpretive practice is always purposive and unavoidably shaped by context. While descriptions of persons and circumstances may ostensibly be offered as objective, factual reports, they nonetheless provide perspectival, if not partisan, versions of the matters described. The details furnished are notable from a particular point of view and are selected for their relevance to the practical purpose for which the description is formulated. Regardless of how much detail is supplied in a description, in theory there is always more information that might be provided. What is included necessarily fails to exhaust all that could be said about a particular referent and is necessarily a purposive selection from what could possibly have been said.

In quasi-adversarial settings like commitment hearings, where partisan interests are at stake, depictions of people and places are understandably shaped and selected with persuasive goals in mind. In such settings, interpretive practice does not convey or report reality as much as it assembles and manages it for the practical purpose at hand. In light of the many disagreements and discrepant interpretations, it is tempting to conclude that participants' descriptions bear no necessary relation to the people and circumstance to whom the descriptions refer. To do so, however, casts participants as nothing more than intentionally disingenuous, calculating rhetoricians—"bad faith" interpreters of the matters at hand.

This is certainly the case in some instances. Nevertheless, the descriptions offered in commitment proceedings are generally no more contrived than those in other everyday situations. Some observations are highlighted, others ignored. Interpretations support preferred conclusions. And it is occasionally obvious that a courtroom participant is offering characterizations that he or she believes are inaccurate. Through tone, posture, and ironic juxtaposition, PDs, DAs, and even judges can distance themselves from their own accounts, interpretations, and descriptions, indicating that what they argued might not match what they "really" observed or believed.

One PD, for example, represented a client whose clothing was dirty, tattered, and disheveled, reeked of urine, and fit so poorly that the man had to constantly clutch and readjust his trousers to keep them from falling off as he stood before the court. By everyday commonsense standards, the man looked terrible. The PD proceeded through a rather routine "defense," culminating in the recommendation that his client should be released. In conclusion, however, he expansively claimed that his client was fully capable of supporting himself while living in the community, ending with, "He's perfectly fit to go looking for a job when he leaves here today." The sarcasm with which the line was delivered clearly conveyed the PD's lack of commitment to the depictions and opinions he had just offered.

Descriptions during commitment hearings, then, are sometimes more explicitly or intentionally rhetorical than others. But it would be both inaccurate and unfair to suggest that interpretive practice was not accountably linked to the objects of interpretation. Almost any characterization could anticipate strenuous challenge, so participants were typically prepared to display the grounds for their claims, providing justificatory accounts that appealed to the "facts" of the case at hand as well as to things that "everybody knows" to be true. Speakers were always accountable for showing how the objects of description were resources for the interpretations offered.

One might argue, however, that partisan interests shape, if not "distort," arguments regarding the objects under consideration, unconsciously if not overtly. But an alternative tack suggests that we analyze conflicting depictions without implying interpretive "bias," focusing instead on the organizational and discursive concerns, constraints, and conventions that condition interpretive practice.

Interpretation is sensitive to social, cultural, and historical context. Visions and versions of social life respond to the interpretive demands, goals, and contingencies of the situation at hand. Descriptions are assembled with reference to preexisting, locally available interpretive templates of the objects of concern. They thus reflect commonly recognized spheres of understanding, local cultures born of shared, repeatedly communicated and routinized interpretive schemes (Gubrium 1991). Particular depictions emerge in conjunction with the social distribution of signs and interpretive structures. Interpretive practice is therefore *organizationally embedded* (Gubrium 1987, 1988; Gubrium and Holstein

1990)—that is, grounded in, and shaped by, the social organization of the domains from which interpretation emerges.[3]

When we encounter contradictory descriptions—for example, the conflicting family depictions in Tom Cline's hearing discussed above— we might understand their divergence in terms of the practical context in which they were assembled. Recall that Dr. Brown claimed that Mr. Cline had "no family to speak of" as he argued for Mr. Cline's commitment. His view, we might argue, oriented to the concerns that constitute his professional and organizational outlook on mental health and illness. Organizational and professional commitments to the therapeutic treatment of mental illness and benevolent guardianship of those unable to fend for themselves provided an interpretive lens for viewing and depicting the circumstances of Mr. Cline's life. As the proposed solution to Mr. Cline's problems, his family appeared therapeutically and custodially inadequate. Dr. Brown expressed this assessment by interpretively denying the domestic character of the household Mr. Cline proposed to occupy; there was "no family to speak of," at least in terms of the way a psychiatrist might conceive of family ties in these circumstances.

Mr. Cline's PD concluded just the opposite—that Mr. Cline indeed had a family whose home was a tenable living option. While clearly rhetorical, her description of his family focused on the security Mr. Cline would experience if he stayed with persons he knew well. In light of her orientation to Mr. Cline's affective well-being and need for a demonstrably supportive environment, the PD accountably depicted the presence of family and its utility as a placement resource. The point here is not that one depiction was more accurate than the other, but that each reflected the interpretive concerns of an organized domain of practical interests. Depictions of age, gender, and other personal and social structures are similarly conditioned by interpretive circumstance, continually providing the possibility for divergent "good faith" portrayals of the same object.

In a sense, as Mary Douglas (1986) puts it, socially organized circumstances come to "think" and "talk" for their participants by providing conventional modes of discourse, practical agendas, and shared interpretive perspectives. This helps account for the ways that interpretive practice yields distinctive, yet accountable constructions—descriptions offered in good faith by interlocutors grounded in alternative circumstances and perspectives. Psychiatrists, judges, PDs, and DAs all orient to particular aspects of their cases, and thus characterize and emphasize aspects of those cases differently, even though their referents may be ostensibly "identical." Organizational embeddedness, then, provides a basis for alternative descriptions of persons, places, and things that speak to the practical, organizationally relevant concerns of the various participants in commitment proceedings.

Still, we must also remember that interactants are not "judgmental dopes" (Garfinkel 1967) who merely react to circumstances and structural imperatives. Rather, they are constantly interpreting the recognizable features of everyday experience, sifting through cultural instructions, articulating available models with everyday occurrences to construct the coherent social realities they inhabit. While circumstances and local cultural context produce interpretive constraints and supply interpretive resources for accomplishing practical descriptions, organizational embeddedness does not dictate interpretive practice.

Notes

1.   Local accountability structures, however, do constrain person-description. Participants, for example, routinely utilized gender and age as interpretive schemas, but were extremely unlikely to invoke race. We may speculate that this category was not useful within a cultural context that discourages explicit public racial "stereotyping," even if racial typifications implicitly exist.

2.   Indeed, the discourse of home and family is frequently employed to address issues of care, concern, custody, and permanence in myriad everyday circumstances unrelated to commitment proceedings (Gubrium and Holstein 1990).

3.   I use the term "organizational" here in its most general sense, referring to any socially structured circumstance. While my examples are drawn from formal organizations, the analysis would also apply to circumstances organized along different lines, say by reference to gender or race. The point is that alternative contexts serve to realize different interpretations according to their varied interpretive options, constraints, and agendas.

Chapter 9

"Action That Divides"

Designating the internment of "madness" as an "act of sovereign reason" by which "men confine their neighbors," Foucault offers a provocative point of departure for analyzing contemporary involuntary commitment proceedings.[1] As a counterhistory of mental illness and psychiatry, *Madness and Civilization*'s central argument is that the formulation of mental illness as a psychiatric condition did not precipitate the separation of the mad from the sane. Rather, Foucault argues, the formulation of the category mental illness and its enforced confinement were reflexively related; eighteenth-century asylums furnished an institutional environment for psychiatry to emerge and were essential to the formulation of modern interpretations of madness, while the development of psychiatric discourse and gaze justified the asylums. Sites of internment and the will to discriminate experience elicited interpretive practices and structures through which the "insane" were separated from the "sane." The mental illness label has become increasingly important as an instrument of this separation. While today's commitment proceedings are not primarily concerned with discerning and judging psychiatric condition, they nonetheless call upon practical reason and commonsense theories about mental illness, community living arrangements, and culturally normal forms to divide some persons from others.

These dividing practices are noteworthy in two major respects. First, interpretive practice in commitment proceedings is *interactional*. The persons and situations under consideration are produced, organized, and assessed through the discursive structures and routines of commitment hearings; claims, arguments, and decisions are conversational projects, orderly talk purposefully assembled in a distinctive institutional environment. Facts are not revealed so much as they are descriptively accomplished. The law does not dictate or control the proceedings as much as it is *used* interactionally to account for claims that are made. As

Miller (1990) argues of human service organizations more generally, the realities upon which participants in commitment proceedings act are the products of rhetorical interpretive practice.

Second, while it is profoundly interactional, interpretation is also *structured*. Interpretive practice organizes our understanding of actions, objects, and circumstances, but practice is itself conditioned by circumstance. Consequently, interpretation reflects its context. Local culture and institutionalized ways of understanding and talking shape the interactions that constitute commitment proceedings. The proceedings' organized context provides interpretive structures to which participants and their talk must orient; the court produces an interactional order for its transactions that is deeply implicated in hearing outcomes.

But interpretive practice is not dictated by context or culture. As Gubrium (1988) suggests, collective representations (Durkheim 1961), social forms, and shared meanings are available for interpretive work, but they must be locally articulated with instances of lived experience. Interpretive practice thus attaches and secures public images and institutionalized discourses to the concrete cases where involuntary commitment is at issue. Commitment proceedings are socially organized occasions for constructing and managing practical realities and enacting cultural forms. Culturally grounded interpretive practice thus underpins the "action that divides."

Mental Illness and Community Custody

Because mental illness has become a necessary but not sufficient warrant for involuntary hospitalization, commitment proceedings focus primarily on how patients might manage practical everyday affairs. Mental status recedes to the interpretive background as nonpsychiatric criteria become paramount. While the relative importance of mental condition was the crux of the labeling theory debate of the 1960s and 1970s—articulated in an overly simplistic and theoretically compromised fashion—the observation that psychiatric criteria do not determine commitment decisions should not be construed as support for either side in that controversy.

Perhaps the presence or absence of symptoms of what might be called mental illness was the critical issue for internment decisions in the times about which Foucault, Scheff, or Gove wrote, but today the issue is all but moot for commitment proceedings. This is not because mental illness is unimportant, but because it is nonproblematic. From the standpoint of participants, everyone sought to be committed is mentally ill. This is the practical reality that commitment proceedings address, confirmed by psychiatric opinion and underscored by deeply rooted assumptions about the conditions and circumstances that propel persons into commitment hearings. While few assume that all of these persons should be hospitalized, everyone involved in commitment hearings believes they are "crazy." Consequently, psychiatric condition per se cannot be used to discriminate between patients. Moreover, trying to predict outcomes of commitment cases based on some imported standard of psychological disturbance or health would be fruitless.[2]

If mental illness is relevant, however, its importance derives from its use as an interpretive framework. Assessments of a patient's conduct and circumstances are reflexively tied to the underlying assumption about what type of person he or she is—that is, a mentally ill person. Mental illness is thus a resource for describing and evaluating the people and situations around which commitment hearings center. The crucial issue is how commonsense notions about mental illness are *used* to understand and interpret the "facts" of commitment cases. The importance of commonsense labeling is far-reaching, but the labeling process should not be understood as either correctly corresponding with or incorrectly contradicting the "reality" of psychiatric condition. Rather, labeling is the process through which psychiatric reality is *constituted* for the practical purpose at hand, and does not rely upon the accuracy of correspondence for its commonsense meaning. To paraphrase W. I. Thomas (1931), if labels are thought to be accurate—thus "real"—they are real in their consequence. Therefore, analyses of the commitment process should examine the ways that labels are employed, and to what effect, instead of attempting to assess their accuracy based on some putatively objective standard derived from outside the situation being examined.[3]

The relevance of this book to the labeling controversy, then, is not that mental illness is unimportant, nor that labeling fails to correspond to "true" psychiatric condition. Rather, the point is that it is analytically unimportant to establish whether or not something objectively knowable as a person's "true psychiatric condition" really exists. According to the practical reasoning exhibited in commitment proceedings, persons have psychiatric conditions, and the conditions of persons sought to be committed are universally pathological. *For participants,* mental illness exists, is real, and has distinct meanings, consequences, and implications. Analysis of labeling or categorization practices should avoid "arguing with the participants" over the correctness of their labeling practices, and focus instead on the ways they engage in commonsense interpretive procedures that utilize labels to produce reasonable arguments and warranted decisions.

From this point of view, the consequences of mental illness assumptions are most apparent—and sometimes commonsensically ironic—in they ways they condition and structure participants' interpretations of patients' testimony, behavior, and community living arrangements. Since arguments for release appear most warranted when a patient (or his or her attorney) convincingly argues that he or she intends to live in a community situation that can accommodate and contain a person *who is mentally ill,* a tenable living situation is one that approximates the structured and encompassing institutionalized setting represented by the mental hospital. This seemingly inverts the logic and implementation of "deinstitutionalized" mental health care that undergirds most reformed commitment legislation.

The community mental health movement has attempted to replace dehumanizing total institutions (Goffman 1961)—which isolate mental patients from nearly all social contact and reinforce passive and dependent behavior patterns—with more natural, therapeutic community settings. This, it is argued, integrates patients with their neighbors, establishes social ties with normal society, and nurtures initiative, responsibility, and independent living skills. In theory, improvement is abetted by circumstances that approximate patients' natural living arrangements. Deinstitutionalization thus aims to capitalize on a wide range of healthful influences thought to inhere in community life (Kirk and Thierren 1975).

But because commitment proceedings orient to participants' distinctive assumptions about mental illness and attendant tenability concerns, claims that depict patients' proposed living arrangements in the terms idealized by the deinstitutionalization movement are susceptible to challenge. And they appear to be less persuasive than arguments contending that highly structured circumstances are available for patients to occupy. That is, patients arguing for release into community circumstances that require and/or promote independent living skills or normal social functioning often find their arguments treated as unreasonable and unwarranted; such circumstances are considered untenable "for mentally ill persons." In contrast, arguments indicating that a patient will be dependent upon other persons and institutions to supervise all aspects of daily life are more likely to meet with favorable reactions because they better address the court's tenability concerns.

The persistent belief in patients' mental illness thus minimizes the likelihood that a person with the desire and opportunity to live in circumstances requiring initiative, responsibility, and control—a conventional living arrangement by most standards—will be allowed to do so. This results in the paradoxical realization that the interpretive environment of commitment hearings militates against the release of those persons who argue that they are capable of living independently in community settings. Conversely, commitment hearings are most receptive to arguments for release that locate patients in neocustodial treatment settings.

Commitment proceedings thus promote a system of "community custody" (Scull 1981) whereby patients must agree to be monitored and supervised, even when they are released. This, in effect, "transinstitutionalizes" both treatment and social control (Warren 1981), requiring that community settings constrain and control the havoc-wreaking symptoms of mental illness that are assumed to follow released patients into their lives beyond the hospital. Thus, mental health care is often "deinstitutionalized" in name alone, as the return of patients to the community extends "the philosophy of custodialism into the community rather than ending it at the gates of the state hospital" (Kirk and Thierren 1975, p. 212).

Accountability Structures

Because commitment proceedings do not discriminate between cases on the basis of mental illness as much as on practical circumstance, interpretive practice orients to a variety of nonpsychiatric standards of accountability. Mental illness remains an important definitional resource for making sense of interpretively enigmatic affect, claims, and behavior, as well as a partial warrant for confining persons who are dangerous or disruptive. But it is only one of several categories that are so implicated. Commitment proceedings ultimately "institutionalize" a related set of concerns—that is, make them salient and routine—to which arguments and decisions must orient. The concerns form a tripartite accountability structure that conditions, if not dictates, commitment proceedings.

Three distinct but interrelated matters organize and channel commitment arguments, providing an interpretive grid to which participants hold one another's claims accountable. To be viable, arguments must display an orientation to and appreciation for each of the following: (1) local interpretations of mental health and illness, (2) cultural images, icons, and normal forms, and (3) compassion, care, and custody for those in need. Arguments failing to address any of the concerns invite challenges to their medical, legal, and/or moral worthiness.

Local Interpretations of Craziness

Concerns about mental illness clearly insinuate most aspects of commitment arguments in fairly standard ways, across cases and jurisdictions. The assumption that patients are mentally ill is invariant, as are claims that the condition is chronic, persistent, potentially debilitating, and requires some sort of intervention. Commitment proceedings are thus accountable to relatively consistent and stable images of mental illness, and tend to articulate these images similarly in the diverse sites studied.

Local variations in how craziness is apprehended, represented, and responded to, however, do exist, demanding local acknowledgment. For example, while criteria for mental health are different for men and women, the particulars and their implications may vary from jurisdiction to jurisdiction. In the isolated rural region served by Northern Court, for instance, "cabin fever"—confinement indoors during the long harsh winters—was said to exacerbate psychiatric distress.[4] This was argued to be an acute problem for women, given their assumed domestic role and generally "social" nature. A woman who "cracked up" under the pressures of winter, it was argued, would become a severe burden on her family, and would likely destroy the household and family if left untreated. Men, while equally subject to the ravages of isolation and confinement, were said to be less affected because the masculine way of exhibiting derangement was typically to disappear into the woods until the problem was "out of his system." This might endanger a man (although men were expected to be able to survive on their own under such circumstances), but he would not pose any threat to the community by making a hermit of himself, or even leaving the area. However, if a deranged man "brought his troubles to town," he would be a likely target for immediate commitment.

The point is not that mental illness has objectively different forms or effects from community to community. Rather, it is that commitment arguments must acknowledge "local cultures of craziness" in order to be accountable and persuasive. While they are variations on a common theme, local interpretations place the demands of mental illness in the context of the immediate social, cultural, and material environment. The diversity of the community served by Metropolitan Court, for example, provided a strikingly variegated cultural backdrop against which conduct and living circumstances were articulated, an interpretive milieu vastly different from those considered in, say, Northern or Southern Court, which occupied traditionally "rural" regions. At the same time, experience with the substantial American Indian population living in the vicinity of Northern Court provided an alternative set of cultural standards and expectations that might influence commitment arguments in ways not found in other jurisdictions.

Local experience within the commitment process itself also conditions interpretive practice. Indeed, individual courtrooms develop their own local cultures of craziness as well as locally institutionalized interpretive and decision-making practices. Metropolitan Court, for example, dealt exclusively with mental health–related cases. Mental patients filled the courtrooms, hallways, and gathering areas every day. Court personnel thus developed a "tolerance" for—even an appreciation of—a range of behaviors that might seem totally bizarre and unsettling to those unfamiliar with the scene. As a particular case was considered against the background of this typical caseload, the distinguishing effects of florid symptoms, outrageous claims, and the like were relatively subdued. Normative standards of conduct and comportment in Metropolitan Court emerged from unrelenting, day-to-day experience with arguably some of the "craziest" members of a community known worldwide for its often outlandish citizenry; compared to the stream of cases running through the courtroom, an individual case had to be "extreme" in some important regard for it to draw any special notice. Conversely, in jurisdictions where commitment cases comprised only a small portion of a court's caseload, standards of and toleration for craziness were different; claims about or displays of mental "symptoms" might command more central positions in commitment arguments. The standards for what constituted an extreme instance of derangement thus varied according to organizational expectations (Emerson 1983).[5]

Cultural Images and Normal Forms

As Chapter 8 has argued, cultural images—working models of reality—and normal forms—known-in-common types of persons and settings—are used as interpretive resources for commitment proceedings. Arguments acquire their reasoned appearance and bolster their persuasiveness by appealing to cultural standards. Images of known types of persons and places are invoked to serve as exemplars for comparison or violation, positing what is acceptable, and by way of contrast, what is inappropriate. Commitment participants offer descriptions of persons of particular genders or age groups, for example, supporting their arguments by referencing gender- or age-typical images. Similarly, images of home and family provide standards of normative accountability for arguments regarding tenable living situations.

Commitment proceedings rely upon cultural themes, but a relatively limited range of forms and images is regularly invoked. Myriad others that might potentially be used are ignored. For example, patients are routinely compared to standards for their age groups or genders, but racial imagery was seldom invoked for comparative purposes. Metropolitan Court has a multiracial clientele, hearing the cases of many African Americans, Hispanics, Middle Easterners, and Asians. Whereas many of these persons were described in terms relating their conduct to the expected behavior of members of their genders or age groups, seldom was race or ethnicity mentioned. This is especially true for African Americans. Cases involving a foreign-born person might elicit references to the person's native culture, but there was never any discussion of American black culture or normative expectations. Occasionally, participants referred to the positive "family values" characteristic of particular ethnic (Hispanics) or religious (Catholics) groups, but racial typing was generally avoided.

The relative absence of the discourse of race from commitment proceedings suggests that the use of racial standards is organizationally inappropriate. Clearly, American culture abounds with racial stereotypes, yet their public use in the context of commitment hearings appears to be taboo, evidently inhibited by local custom and practiced aversion. There are, of course, exceptions. Commonsense theories about American Indians were occasionally used in Northern Court, for example. But, in general, race is absent from the publicly displayed interpretive orientations of commitment proceedings.

Commitment arguments, then, produce locally relevant aspects of American culture to interpret the particulars of individual cases. They make visible those institutions and characteristics about which there seems to be widespread cultural agreement. Observers of commitment proceeding thus have displayed for them cultural ideals of what it means to be male or female, old or young, crazy or sane. Proceedings offer standards of domesticity, images of a proper home and family life. While there is no formal or predictable way of invoking the images, their use reproduces normal American culture in the process of designating aberrant and disruptive elements. Hearing participants articulate what is "normal" as they formulate problems of deviation.[6] Commitment arguments are critically accountable to "what everyone knows" to be true about contemporary life in the communities in which commitment proceedings take place.

Compassion, Care, and Custody

Tenability arguments are the most prominent manifestations of a pervasive desire for commitment proceedings to be compassionate toward the plight of mental patients. Merely displaying sympathetic attitudes, however, is insufficient, for compassion must also be enacted through arrangements for guardianship—sometimes formal, but often loosely and informally construed—and community care. While care and custody have clear implications for maintaining community order, their central importance to public commitment arguments is as a "configuration of concern" (Gubrium and Holstein 1990) expressing participants' orientation to patients' well-being. Arguments must sustain this focus or endanger their accountability.

As tenability arguments concentrate on community living circumstances, they often call upon the virtually unassailable, salutary image of family life (Gubrium and Holstein 1990) to address the configuration of concern. Arguments draw upon generally shared notions of what a home or a family is like in order to establish that a proposed placement—either in or outside the hospital—is properly caring, hence, a viable release option. Domestic imagery is used to convey commonsense understandings about what constitutes compassionate care and guardianship. Participants routinely offer the home as a superior alternative to hospitalization, arguing that home care is the prototype for deinstitutionalization, providing superior services without depersonalization or deprivation. Similarly, hospitalization arguments may point to the "homelike" qualities of institutionalized care, or note the absence of home or family from the proposed community arrangements. Domestic discourse thus provides a way of interpreting and conveying contemporary ideals of mental health care. Indeed, in the context of arguments against hospitalization, home and family discourse invokes a descriptive culture of deinstitutionalization, with "home care" as the paragon of *community* mental health care.

The discourses of home and family confront the configuration of concern, addressing issues of patient management, accommodations, and therapy, as well as affective tone, devotion, intimacy, and responsibility. As collective representations, images of home and family encourage us to attach their diverse components to one another, summoning one as we invoke any of the others, especially as they relate to the configuration of concern. Thus, common and tacit assumptions about home care are consolidated in its descriptive usage, implicitly addressing tenability concerns through domestic descriptions. To say that a patient would benefit from being placed "in the home" imparts assurances of security, familiarity, devotion, and so on, clearly expressing compassion and concern for the patient while invoking the ideals of deinstitutionalization.

Of course, organizational embeddedness provides hearing participants with distinctive ways of interpreting home and family, institutionalized incitements to depict and hear domestic experience in particular terms that address the practical issues at hand (Gubrium 1992). And despite the ways that it may be tied to organizational location and collective representations, one's accountability to the configuration of concern is nonetheless artfully manifested, awaiting occasions of practical interpretive activity for its display.

Accountability and the Law

Commitment proceedings are most explicitly accountable to legal statutes. While the law ostensibly dictates procedures and criteria for arguing and deciding cases, actual proceedings are not rigidly bound procedurally or substantively to a prespecified format. Indeed, commitment
laws may best be analyzed as accounting resources rather than directives
for conduct. Laws do not, in and of themselves, dictate or constrain
behavior. Their application to concrete occurrences may provide the
warrant for sanctions, but the mere existence of laws guarantees neither
compliance nor enforcement. We are, however, respectful of laws in the
sense that we typically fashion our conduct so that compliance with the
law is demonstrable, if we are called into account. Commitment arguments respond to the law in this fashion.

Hearing participants fortify their arguments by showing how they
accord with or are compelled by the law. As in other legal settings,
displaying the reasoned, principled, and legal character of an account,
recommendation, or explanation is likely to make it more persuasive
(Holstein 1983). Competent, accountable arguments display how they
comply with or are compelled by the law; legitimate arguments and
decisions are demonstrably legal. Commitment statutes are rhetorical
assets and should therefore be analyzed in terms of *rule use* (Zimmerman
1970) rather than rule following.

While the law is neither an a priori restraint, nor a prescription for
arguments and decisions, it is nonetheless a commanding orientation.
Court personnel anticipate that their claims will be held accountable to
the law, so they produce arguments that can be legally justified. The law,
of course, is broadly interpretable—not a fixed rubric, but a situationally
formulated and invoked set of guidelines. As they invoke commitment
statutes to justify their arguments, hearing participants articulate the
law's relevance to matters as hand, producing the specifics of an abstract, open-ended code. Invoking the law, then, is an interpretive practice for rendering arguments accountable, thus rhetorically compelling.[7]

Rationalizing Compassion, Domesticating Control

The interactional framework of commitment proceedings keeps accountability at the forefront; claims and explanations can always be
contested. While the interpretive production of the "realities" of commitment cases might appear somewhat insubstantial, evanescent, or
arbitrary (indeed, some might say contrived), the demand for accounta-

bility requires that these realities evince a practical concreteness that can withstand interpretive challenge. Commitment laws and procedures provide a rhetorical scaffold upon which arguments and claims may be suspended. Commitment arguments must also display compassion and promise care for persons who hospitalization is under consideration. The commitment process encourages arguments and decisions that legally, accountably enact the configuration of concerns for the psychiatrically deranged.

Indeed, commitment proceedings might be framed as a contemporary "rationalization" of compassion. According to Giddens (1979), rationalization is the process of explaining why we act as we do by giving reasons for our conduct. We rationalize action by attaching purposes, goals, and motives to conduct to display its apparent reasonableness.[8] Providing motives or reasons for action rationalizes it, making it a meaningful and understandable feature of everyday life. Commitment proceedings thus rationalize the confinement of selected persons by showing how detention and care result from the court's organized expression of compassion.

But there is another sense in which compassion is rationalized. Max Weber referred to "formal rationality" as the organization of conduct according to calculated principles, formal rules, and institutionalized procedures (Weber 1958, 1968). Rationalized social relations are organized so that they accord with general principles, promoting the predictability to which modern organizations and bureaucracies aspire. Following this usage, commitment proceeding are bureaucratic manifestations of the desire to rationalize compassionate intervention.

Commitment laws and procedures formalize the community's concern for the mentally ill, providing a standard format for imposing care and custody. The abstract notion of legally mandated involuntary commitment transforms decisions to care and confine from private, individual matters usually involving family and close associates into public, institutional obligations for dispassionate agents of the community at large. Concretely, the community is charged with the responsibility of caring for its unfortunate members and is provided with the rational, bureaucratic apparatus to implement this care.

While the transformation provides some assurance that troubled and troublesome community members will receive attention, it also depersonalizes compassion and concern. As Weber noted, the more fully rationalized an organization becomes, "the more completely it succeeds in eliminating from official business love, hatred, and all purely personal, irrational, and emotional elements" (Weber 1968, p. 975). Rationalization thus contravenes and subordinates some of the most distinctive values of western culture—creativity, spontaneity, and individual autonomy

(Giddens 1971)—diminishing the import and appropriateness of nonrational factors like intuition, sentiment, and emotion.

In addition, rationalization takes the form of an increasing reliance upon expert knowledge and authority—especially scientific expertise. This leads to the embodiment of that expertise in organizational structure and guidelines so that participants cease to think and act in "human" (and humane) ways, but merely follow general procedures. Decision-making and conduct abandon personal, human control in service to organizational agendas. Borrowing from Weber, the life world is "disenchanted" in that there is no space, no role left for personalized, spontaneous thought and action. Indeed, Weber feared that rationalization might ultimately deny its participants the essence of their humanity (Giddens 1971), "parcelling-out" their souls (Bendix 1960) in the calculated, efficient pursuit of goals. Abstract laws and formal procedures, it appears, may eliminate some forms of arbitrariness, but in exchange they introduce an impersonal monopoly over how compassion, concern, and control are asserted into people's lives.

If rationalizing compassion restricts the humanity of commitment decision-making, however, the situated, artful nature of interpretive practice reasserts human agency. As Gubrium (1992) argues, organizationally embedded rationalization is neither uniform nor totalized, but is diversely constituted through rationality's local interpretive machineries and images. Rationalization is diverse, reflecting individual authorship as well as the influence of various domains of interpretive practice. This is evident, for example, in the myriad ways that commitment laws may be invoked, and the innumerable factors that can be considered as commitment cases are argued.

Despite their reliance upon formal, legal formulas, commitment proceedings are also receptive to other forms of practical reasoning. As something of a counterbalance to the rationalization of compassion, for example, recommendations for commitment are often rendered accountable by reference to the deeply personal, sentimental images of home and family. Put differently, these arguments "domesticate" care, confinement, and control, using culturally shared idealizations of family life to convey the salutary character of recommended placement options, including institutional alternatives.

As Chapter 8 suggests, arguments favoring confinement are particularly noteworthy for the ways that family discourse and domestic imagery are used to display the caring, restorative aspects of environments into which mentally troubled persons are committed. The family rhetoric reasserts some of the compassion and concern for individual's affective well-being that are inevitably overshadowed as one argues for any form of enforced detention. In addition, "family responsibility" may be invoked as an obligation of the state in order to justify coercive actions, offering a rationale for acting in the disturbed person's "best interest," even when that person strenuously objects. A case involving a homeless person and the city of New York is both illustrative and notorious in this regard.[9]

In the mid-1980s, New York City instituted a program called Project Help. Field teams, comprised of nurses, social workers, and psychiatrists, were deployed to identify and monitor the homeless with mental problems, providing them with needed food, clothing, and medical care. If, in the team's opinion, an individual appeared to be an immediate threat to him- or herself or others, or a threat in the "foreseeable future," they assisted in committing the person to a mental hospital, involuntarily if necessary.

In 1988, the city was embroiled in a controversy surrounding the involuntary commitment of a forty-year-old African American woman named Joyce Brown. Ms. Brown had been living on the streets of Manhattan's Upper East Side, homeless, without any stable source of income, but refusing to take refuge in any of the city's shelters for the homeless and indigent. She had a history of psychiatric problems and some casual observers indicated that she was deranged, abusive, and would accost and annoy people on the streets. Others reported that she behaved as a perfectly personable, rational woman.

Citing commitment statutes, the city had Ms. Brown admitted to a special psychiatric ward at Bellvue Hospital, where city psychiatrists diagnosed her as a delusional paranoid schizophrenic. She strenuously objected to the commitment, however, and engaged the services of American Civil Liberties Union (ACLU) attorneys to fight the commitment in a formal hearing before a judge. The attorneys argued that Ms. Brown was intelligent, coherent, and articulate, and could take care of herself; she didn't need to be hospitalized. Ms. Brown rationally explained some of her "bizarre" behaviors, like burning money given to her by passersby, defecating in the streets, and refusing to go to overnight shelters because they were too dangerous. Three psychiatrists testified that Ms. Brown was not mentally ill. One of Ms. Brown's attorneys concluded with a classic "tenability" argument:

> She has a track record of living on the street for over a year, keeping herself warm, providing food for herself, entering the hospital in good physical condition. A person like that simply doesn't meet the civil commitment standards under the Constitution or under existing law. (CBS Television, *60 Minutes*, January 24, 1988)

The judge terminated Ms. Brown's commitment, but the city appealed and won. Ms. Brown was readmitted to Bellvue, where she filed an appeal. Subsequently, the city released Ms. Brown when she agreed to stay in a hotel where counselors were available to help her.

Several times over the course of the proceedings, New York Mayor Ed Koch articulated the city's concerns, each time seeking to justify the city's intransigence about confining and treating a woman who was arguably doing no serious harm to herself or others. He stated the following, for example:

> It is terrible to see these people who are lying in their own feces, who are clearly gross mental cases, who if they were your mother or sister or a family relative you would want to pick up and take to a hospital right away, even if they resisted, because they are mentally incompetent to make such a judgment. . . . We're doing exactly what her family would do for her, but in this case her family happens to be the city of New York. (*60 Minutes*, January 24, 1988)

Ms. Brown, of course, disagreed. When asked about living the street, for instance, she replied:

> If that's . . . the way the person wants to live their life, and they're an adult, who am I to say that they can't do that? Now if the person's committing a crime, that's a different story. But if they're just sitting on the street, dirty and nasty, that's not a crime. . . . In a civilized society, you just don't go around picking up people against their will and bringing them to the hospital when they're sane, just because of a mayor's program. All of this is political. I am a political prisoner because of Mayor Koch. (*60 Minutes*, January 24, 1988)

The political agenda, Ms. Brown's lawyer argued, was to remove a poor person who "didn't belong there" from the streets of a fashionable neighborhood. The city, he claimed, was motivated not by compassion but by the desire to keep the unsightly out of sight.

Asking a question Foucault might have formulated, *60 Minutes* interviewer Morley Safer asked Mayor Koch, "Don't you have some qualms about using the law in which psychiatry is used to deprive someone of their liberty?" Koch replied:

> There's no reason in the world for the city of New York to hold her against her will except for the fact that we don't want her lying in her feces on the sidewalk, not because it offends people who pass by, but because it's compassionate. (*60 Minutes*, January 24, 1988)

At issue throughout this case was the city's unsolicited intervention into the life of a citizen whose choices regarding material support, domicile, and life-style were unconventional. While Ms. Brown argued that the city's interest was coercive and political, the city countered with paternalism, expressly framing its actions as those of a concerned family. In the words of Mayor Koch, the city was only doing for Joyce Brown "exactly what her family would do for her." Indeed, from the mayor's perspective, the city was Ms. Brown's surrogate, if not actual, family. And it assumed familial responsibility not out of disgust, politics, or self-interest, but "because it's compassionate"—what any family member would do for another member because of the bond of caring.

Simultaneously describing and rationalizing the city's "compassion," Koch transformed the putatively coercive aspects of the city's intervention into familial benevolence. His family rhetoric provided a literal realization of the doctrine of *parens patriae*, reflexively establishing the government's responsibility to act as a concerned "parent" to its citizens while reconstituting the city as Ms. Brown's family by virtue of its care and concern. In effect, he "domesticated" the control being exercised, blunting its coercive edge with familial kindness and good will.

The process of "domestication" is so prevalent in commitment proceedings that cases sometimes sound like virtual debates over the social problem of homelessness acted out on the small stage of individual lives. In perhaps its most simple representation, tenability is equated with a living situation's "homelike" qualities; grave disability can be conflated with having no home and no family to turn to—that is, homelessness. To the extent that one is described as homeless during commitment proceedings, one is vulnerable to being hospitalized *for one's own good*. Written large, the response suggests that the problem of the homeless mentally ill—who are naively presumed to comprise a massive segment of America's homeless population (Snow, Baker, Anderson, and Martin 1986)—is appropriately addressed through domesticated institutionalization, that is, by providing surrogate "homes" for the troubled and dispossessed. As we noted in the previous discussion of community custody, this offer ironically twists the realization, if not the goals, of deinstitutionalized mental health care. It also raises the haunting prospect, adumbrated in Joyce Brown's case, of the state seeking to remedy problems with persons who reject or who are unable to attain conventional life-styles and living accommodations by attaching psychiatric labels and imposing paternalistic confinement.[10]

Commitment proceedings thus rationalize compassion and domesticate control. In the process, their interactional matrix of interpretive practices supplies the machinery for expressing social problems and their solutions in culturally viable terms. Those terms, however, promote preferred psychiatric understandings of intra- and interpersonal difficulties, sometimes obscuring what some argue are unwarranted deprivations of liberty (Morse 1982). Is involuntary commitment, then, "another form of madness"? The question is not simply answered.

Commitment proceeding are eminently reasoned, and conscientiously orient to the law. They enact culturally grounded moral values in procedurally governed circumstances. But the sane and insane, or the normal and incompetent, are not simply discerned and separated; rather, they are socially constructed in cultural and institutional context. Descriptions and claims become "true" or "accurate" not by virtue of their correspondence to objective reality, but through the local conventions of interpretive practice. The value of the goals sanctioned by the law and the legitimacy of culturally promoted accountability structures are not issues for sociological adjudication; they are political, philosophical, ethical questions relating to issues of responsibility, care, control, and personal liberty. But the interpretive practices that enact culture and enforce goals are eminently social; the practical reasoning through which courtroom realities are fashioned, and upon which commitment decisions are based, invites sociological description, if not endorsement. To understand how some persons are committed and others go free requires an appreciation of the social process through which "court-ordered insanity"—institutionally organized interpretations of mental illness and its consequences—is used to manifest the compassion, care, and control implied by the ideals of involuntary commitment.

Notes

1.   And while the characterization of acts of confinement as "that other form of madness" is arguable, it raises several extremely problematic issues. First, of course, is the definition of madness that Foucault seeks to employ. As Derrida and others have noted, Foucault relies upon representations of madness that strive to transcend the relation between language and the objects it seeks to represent, perpetrating the same sorts of "exclusions" that Foucault himself denounces in *Madness and Civilization* (Felman 1985). A second set of issues relates to the definition and evaluation of confinement and commitment—that is, whether they are forms of repression replete with violent silencing, or something else, perhaps more compassionate, if not liberating or empowering.
2.   This was, of course, the tactic employed in the labeling theory debate, and no doubt contributed to the failure to resolve it.
3.   There has been a kind of analytic absurdity in the competing analyses of commitment proceedings and labeling practices. Various studies have attempted to independently evaluate the psychiatric condition of candidate patients, but they did so *outside* the context of actual commitment proceedings. Dispassionate, disinterested observers provided evaluations, but as "academic" or "theoretical" exercises. The evaluations were not subject to the practical orientations that conditioned actual commitment hearing participants' assessments, and were thus operating upon a phenomenal reality distinctly different from that comprised by actual commitment proceedings.
4.   Local lore held that a well-adjusted person learned to cope with the

winters as a way of life, but that psychiatric frailties were likely to be aggravated into full-blown disturbances by the long months of isolation and confinement. Hence, "cabin fever" did not precisely "drive people crazy," but merely hastened the deterioration of those persons inclined to psychiatric problems.

5. Encounters with florid symptoms were everyday fare in Metropolitan Court, and were relatively uncommon in Northern and Southern Courts. The other courts studied saw commitment cases on a routine basis, but they were not devoted solely to commitment hearings. Eastern Court, for example, was located in a community that was home to several major psychiatric wards as well as a state mental health facility. So while mental patients might differ from criminal or civil litigants most often seen in court, their presence was sufficiently common that court personnel were quite accustomed to most of their special features. In any case, and despite the variation in the "appreciation" for patient's troubles and "tolerance" of their behaviors, commitment proceedings never treated mental illness as their predominant criterion for hospitalization.

6. Commitment proceedings might be considered boundary-maintaining occasions. It would be more precise, however, to say that the proceedings constitute, rather than discover or maintain, boundaries. They produce on each occasion those interpretive regions that are bounded, as well as their line of demarcation.

7. This perspective on the law has practical implications for social policy- and lawmaking. If law does not compel behavior, but is instead a sort of accountability framework or resource for argumentation, this should be taken into consideration as legislation is revised and reformed. Revised legislation may offer different accountability structures and rhetorical resources. Therefore, any effort to alter the law should consider its ultimate objective, then anticipate how the reformulated statutes might be used—by persons interactionally invoking and enforcing the law—to achieve the objective. While revised commitment law cannot enforce compliance, it may realign participants' orientation to the commitment process, and be available in some new fashion as an open-ended resource for sanctioned argument.

8. Giddens's usage is similar to Garfinkel's use of the term "account-able." By this Garfinkel means procedures through which social actions are brought to adequate description (Heritage 1984).

9. This case was reported in such high-profile national media outlets as televison's *60 Minutes* and *The Phil Donahue Show,* as well as *The New York Times* and *Los Angeles Times* news services, and ABC's, CBS's, and NBC's nightly news programs. See Campbell and Reeves (1989) for a discussion of the news media's portrayal of the Joyce Brown story.

10. There is ample precedent for such a movement. The theory and practice of juvenile justice in the 1800s, for example, attempted to "domesticate" the treatment of juvenile's in a strikingly similar fashion. Just as today's commitment proceedings assume candidate patients' mental illness, juveniles came to be seen as malleable individuals who could be shaped, and thus saved, by benevolent treatment. First by abandoning the "house of refuge" in favor of the "family reform school"—complete with surrogate parents—then later by using the juvenile court and probation system to "fix the families" of troubled youth, the American justice system relied upon many of the same accounts that are currently used to justify involuntary commitment (Schlossman 1977).

Appendices

The following appendices contain complete transcriptions of three commitment hearings conducted in Metropolitan Court. Transcriptions were done according to the procedures and transcription conventions outlined in Chapters 2 and 5. The cases are selected to illustrate the range of conversational activities and topics that characterize commitment hearings. While they are typical in many respects, these hearings are not intended to represent all hearings; they are neither model nor modal hearings.

Appendix 1:   Patient Polly Brown

[Twenty-five- to thirty-year-old African American, dressed in flowered house coat with red bandanna headband]

[Metropolitan Court; J1, DA4, PD2, Dr16]

1.	J1:	Can we get started with Brown Mr. Perez?
2.	DA4:	All set your honor. Call Dr. Coleman. [Witness occupies
3.		witness stand.]
4.	J1:	I'll remind you that you're still under oath. [The witness
5.		had been sworn in for an earlier hearing.]
6.	DA4:	Please state your name.
7.	Dr16:	Terrance Coleman.
8.	DA4:	[spoken to PD2] Will counsel stipulate to Dr. Coleman's
9.		qualifications?
10.	PD2:	Stipulated.
11.	DA4:	Dr. Coleman, are you familiar with the patient?
12.	Dr16:	Yes.
13.	DA4:	Have you interviewed her?
14.	Dr16:	Yes, several times.

15. DA4:   And you've examined her?
16. Dr16: Again on several occasions.
17. DA4:   Have you discussed the case with other staff members?
18. Dr16: Yes.
19. DA4:   Have you reviewed her records?
20. Dr16: Yes, several times.
21. DA4:   And do you have a professional opinion regarding the patient's
22.   mental condition?
23. Dr16: I do.
24. DA4:   And your diagnosis?
25. Dr16: The patient, Ms. Brown, has a bipolar disorder.
26. DA4:   And is the illness serious?
27. Dr16: Quite.
28. DA4:   Why was Ms. Brown brought into the hospital?
29. Dr16: She was brought in by the police. They were called by her
30.   family and they found her on the roof of her home, saying that
31.   she was going to soar off. She had been trying to get her
32.   children to go on the roof with her. (She had been acting very
33.   erratic, moody and unpredictable. She said she was going to do
34.   a number of things that would be harmful to herself and those
35.   around her. She threatened her brother and told him to stay
36.   away from her children.)
37. DA4:   And she's been under treatment for several days now?
38. Dr16: Right.
39. DA4:   Has she been given any medications?
40. Dr16: Yes, but there hasn't been much change.
41. DA4:   And how would you describe her behavior since she's been
42.   hospitalized?
43. Dr16: She's been quite agitated, verbally abusive. Very aggressive
44.   on the ward. She's required restraints to keep her away from
45.   others and has been banging her head on the wall and has had to
46.   be restrained to keep her from hurting herself. (She has been
47.   erratic in her interactions, and difficult for anyone to get
48.   along with. She has threatened staff members and other
49.   patients.)
50. DA4:   Based on your opinion of the patient's mental illness, do you
51.   feel that she is capable of providing for her own food, clothes,
52.   and shelter?
53. Dr16: I don't believe she could. Polly doesn't have any concept of
54.   handling money. She ran up a two-hundred-dollar water bill
55.   taking baths all day and leaving the water running. She spends
56.   large sums on wine, money she can't really afford. She bought
57.   foolish gifts, things she can't afford to be buying. (She
58.   bought gifts like jewelry and clothing for everyone in the
59.   household and for many of her friends at church.) She said
60.   she was going to live in Dallas, said she had a boyfriend there.
61.   (She was very incoherent about where she would live.) She has

62.		been hospitalized about twenty times since 1966, six times in
63.		the last year. Given her history and diagnosis [bipolar
64.		disorder] I have to say that Polly's mental condition makes her
65.		gravely disabled. Due to her mental illness, she has no way
66.		of supporting, looking after herself, no place to live.
67.		She just ends up back in the hospital.
68.	DA4:	Where does she get the money she spends?
69.	Dr16:	Social Security.
70.	DA4:	And what about a place to live? Where does she say she will go?
71.	Dr16:	Dallas. She said she was a (player?) and she had a boyfriend
72.		there. When I talked to her, she was pretty incoherent about
73.		this.
74.	DA4:	Have you spoken to her mother?
75.	Dr16:	Her mother said she didn't want her to come back in her present
76.		condition.
77.	DA4:	Has the patient been hospitalized previously.
78.	Dr16:	Yes, many times. About twenty times since 1966. She's been
79.		hospitalized six times in the last year.
80.	DA4:	I guess that's all. Thank you Dr. Coleman.
81.	J1:	Mr. Webster.
82.	PD2:	You say she's been in the hospital six times in a year?
83.	Dr16:	That's right.
84.	PD2:	And she's been discharged five times?
85.	Dr16:	I suppose.
86.	PD2:	Was she discharged before or after fourteen days?
87.	Dr16:	The last time she stayed five or six days.
88.	PD2:	When was the last time she lived in Dallas?
89.	Dr16:	I really don't know. (She's lived in this area for six years.)
90.		I'm just quoting her when I say Dallas is her home.
91.	PD2:	Where is Ms. Brown currently living?
92.	Dr16:	Presently she lives with her mother and sister.
93.	PD2:	Did you ever see that water bill you mentioned?
94.	Dr16:	No.
95.	PD2:	Does she have a separate meter from the rest of the family?
96.	Dr16:	I don't know about that.
97.	PD2:	Was this a monthly bill? How long was this bill for?
98.	Dr16:	Her mother said it was for one month.
99.	PD2:	Now, how did her mother determine that it was her [Polly] that
100.		ran up this bill?
101.	Dr16:	I don't know. The mother just said // she did.
102.	J1:	((breaking in)) How would she know that?
103.	PD2:	Your honor I'm just trying to establish the fact that there
104.		were several people in the household and if a lot of water was
105.		being used, the others must have been using some of it and it's
106.		not proven that Ms. Brown was responsible for this bill.
107.	J1:	You've made your point, Mr. Webster. Let's continue.
108.	PD2	OK, now does my client buy her food separately from her family?

109.	Dr16:	She gives her Social Security check to her mother, so I don't
110.		think so.
111.	PD2:	You said that in the hospital she has been agitated and been
112.		threatening others. What is the nature of this?
113.	Dr16:	Well, a staff nurse reported to me that she had overheard the
114.		patient threatening another nurse. She claimed the nurse
115.		called her children bastards and she threatened her
116.		[the nurse].
117.		((silence five seconds))
118.	PD2:	That's all I have, thank you doctor.
119.	J1:	[To DA4] So you're proceeding solely on the issue of grave
120.		disability, am I right?
121.	DA4:	That's right, your honor.
122.	J1:	Witness Mr. Webster.
123.	PD2:	Ms. Brown would like to speak your honor.
124.		[Polly Brown is sworn in.]
125.	PD2:	If the judge releases you, Polly, where will you go?
126.	PB:	I'll go with my children. We'll live at my mother's house.
127.	PD2:	Is that OK with her?
128.	PB:	Of course. She's my mother, my family. She won't kick me out
129.		// for a little fussin.
130.	PD2:	((breaking in)) How long have you lived with your mother?
131.	PB:	I've been there approximately three years.
132.	PD2:	Have you ever lived in Dallas?
133.	PB:	I spent the whole summer there.
134.	PD2:	Did you say that you'd move to Dallas if you got out of Metro?
135.	PB:	I'm hoping to go to Dallas someday. Not now. I want to get
136.		away from here eventually. The state of California is crippling
137.		my mind. // But I'm not crazy. I'm fine. I'm intelligent.
138.		I'll go wherever I want.
139.	PD2:	((breaking in)) But you'll go to your mother's first.
140.	PB:	Of course.
141.	PD2:	Is it true that your mother said she doesn't want you to stay
142.		with her any more?
143.	PB:	That's a lie. She said she would take me. She can't come
144.		today, but a friend of mine will pick me up and take me home.
145.		(PD asks several questions regarding Ms. Brown's ability to
146.		provide for her food, clothing, and shelter. Ms. Brown indicates
147.		that she can provide these things.)
148.	PD2:	Are you responsible for a two-hundred-dollar water bill, Polly?
149.	PB:	That's ridiculous. There ain't no two-hundred-dollar bill.
150.	PD2:	Then why did the doctor mention it?
151.	PB:	I don't know. Maybe my mama said so and got confused.
152.	PD2:	OK Polly, that's fine. So do you have anything else you want
153.		to tell the judge?
154.	PB:	No, that's all.
155.	DA4:	((silence ten seconds)) Why were you brought to the hospital,

156.		Ms. Brown?
157.	PB:	I called the police. My brother had been threatening me so I
158.		went out on the roof to get away. (We can walk on the roof.
159.		It has a doorway and a rail. We go there all the time to get
160.		some sun. It's very nice in the morning. I tried to get my
161.		children to come out on the roof with me where they would be
162.		safe from my brother.) I called the police before I went out.
163.	DA4:	Were you going to jump? Did you say you were going to fly away
164.	PB:	I'd jump if I had to. But he [the brother] stopped when the
165.		police got there. (I was just trying to save my kids. I
166.		didn't want to jump but I would if we were in danger. I was
167.		afraid of my brother.)
168.	DA4:	But the police took you to the hospital. Why you?
169.	PB:	I don't know. My mother was confused and she musta told them
170.		I'd gone crazy.
171.	DA4:	((silence five seconds)) What about this water bill? Did you run
172.		it up?
173.	PB:	No sir. I just bathe twice a day. I'm a heavy woman and I
174.		sweat a lot. I have to bathe twice.
175.	DA4:	And did you use the phone to call Dallas?
176.	PB:	Yes, I have called Dallas. I have a boyfriend there.
177.	DA4:	Do you know how much that costs?
178.	PB:	I call at night.
179.	DA4:	Do you pay rent?
180.	PB:	I give my mother $165 to pay rent and the bills. It comes
181.		from my Social Security.
182.	DA4:	That's all your honor. Thank you Ms. Brown.
183.	J1:	Comments Mr. Webster?
184.	PD2:	There's no evidence suggesting that my client is gravely
185.		disabled, your honor, no reason to be hospitalized. She's
186.		shown that she has a place to go //
187.	J1:	((breaking in)) The mother says that's
188.		not so.
189.	PD2:	No your honor that is not fact. That is hearsay that has been
190.		introduced as a basis for the doctor's medical opinion, but
191.		does not contribute evidence on the matter of grave disability.
192.	J1:	Mr. Webster, according to section 801C an expert witness can
193.		rely upon hearsay in the formulation of his professional
194.		opinion. This is admissible // testimony.
195.	PD2:	((breaking in)) It's only admissible as the basis of
196.		his opinion, but it is not established as a fact in the case.
197.		(Most of the facts that the doctor talked about have not been
198.		established. It has not been established who called the police,
199.		who was threatening who, how money had been spent,
200.		if there were large telephone or water bills.) The doctor has
201.		never even seen the two-hundred-dollar water bill. No one is
202.		sure who is responsible for this. When you start looking at his

203.   opinion and pull the cornerstones away from it, when you look at
204.   the pieces of this case it begins to fall apart. (We have shown
205.   that the doctor's opinion is not based on anything that has
206.   been clearly established. He hasn't seen the water bill. It
207.   may have been for several months.) As for providing for
208.   herself, when my client gets her money she hands it directly
209.   over to her mother. Her Social Security check. She has fully
210.   explained her presence on the roof. (She was there to avoid
211.   her brother. It is more like a sun deck than a roof. It's not
212.   a sloping roof. The family goes out on it all the time.) As
213.   for her behavior in the hospital, we have heard that a nurse
214.   called her children bastards. I believe anyone would be
215.   agitated if they heard this sort of talk. She's protective like
216.   any mother would be. Any woman with children would be
217.   upset. ((silence)) There's no proof of grave disability
218.   here. I'll submit it.
219.   J1:   Mr. Perez.
220.   DA4:   Submitted your honor.
221.   ((silence one minute))
222.   J1:   I'm going to grant the writ in this matter. She seems to have
223.   herself pretty well together, and there are some shaky details
224.   to this case, doctor. [spoken to Ms. Brown] You'll go stay
225.   with your mother and let her look after you, right? I'm not
226.   certain that the mother will take her back in but if not,
227.   she'll be right back in the same soup again and we'll get
228.   another crack at this. You can go Ms. Brown.
229.   PB: Thank you judge. [Ms. Brown stands up, walks over to the
230.   doctor and shakes hands with him.]
231.   [Spoken to doctor good-naturedly] You. You tell stories on me.
232.   J1:   OK, who's next?

Appendix 2:   Patient Regina Farmer

[Approximately thirty-year-old African American, dressed in T-shirt
and shorts with a bandanna around her head]

[Metropolitan Court; J2, DA1, PD3, Dr2]

1.   J2:   Next case.
2.   DA1:   Ready, your honor. We'll do Regina Farmer. Can I have Dr.
3.   Fischer? [Witness occupies witness stand and is sworn in.]
4.   DA1:   Please state your name and spell it please.
5.   Dr2:   Arnold Fischer. That's F I S C H E R.
6.   DA1:   What is your occupation?
7.   Dr2:   I'm an M D psychiatrist.
8.   DA1:   Where did you receive your training?

9.	Dr2:	Wilson University Medical School in New York.
10.	DA1:	Are you licensed?
11.	Dr2:	Yes.
12.	DA1:	Certified?
13.	Dr2:	Yes.
14.	DA1:	Where did you do your psychiatric residency?
15.	Dr2:	Stonebrooke Psychiatric.
16.	DA1:	How long have you been practicing psychiatry?
17.	Dr2:	A little over sixteen years.
18.	DA1:	And you are currently practicing?
19.	Dr2:	At Metro State Hospital.
20.	DA1:	How long have you been there?
21.	Dr2:	About seven months.
22.	DA1:	Have you ever testified at a habeas corpus proceeding?
23.	Dr2:	Yes. I've also done commitment hearings in New York.
24.	DA1:	Stipulate to the doctors qualifications?
25.	PD3:	In a minute. Doctor, are you familiar with LPS?
26.	Dr2:	Yes, I've testified on LPS cases in California before.
27.	PD3:	Stipulate to the qualifications.
28.	DA1:	Are you familiar with the patient, doctor?
29.	Dr2:	Yes.
30.	DA1:	Have you examined her?
31.	Dr2:	Yes.
32.	DA1:	Spoken to other staff members about her?
33.	Dr2:	Yes.
34.	DA1:	Reviewed her chart?
35.	Dr2:	Yes.
36.	DA1:	And have your formulated a medical opinion of the patient's
37.		mental status?
38.	Dr2:	My diagnosis is substance abuse, PCP psychosis. In addition
39.		I've diagnosed a bipolar disorder.
40.	DA1:	What fact or facts are the basis for your diagnosis?
41.	Dr2:	I've based it on a series of lab tests and the patient's
42.		behavior. (The patient was brought to the hospital by the
43.		police because she had been hostile and belligerent to
44.		strangers in a public place. She has taken large amounts of
45.		PCP and has been seriously delusional. The lab tests indicate
46.		that she has toxic levels of PCP in her system. It takes quite
47.		a while to get the PCP out of her system.) I wish she would
48.		stay until the PCP abates. She's been very delusional. Says
49.		she was a television star. (She claimed she was the star of a
50.		major TV series but was currently on hiatus from production.)
51.		She has demonstrated consistently poor judgment. When we
52.		asked her what she would do if she had five hundred dollars,
53.		she said that she would buy a television set. She's been assaultive on
54.		the ward, threatening others, being very disruptive. She has poor
55.		reality contact and her mind and talk wander off when she's

56.		asked a question.
57.	DA1:	In your opinion is the patient gravely disabled, that is,
58.		unable to provide for food, clothing, and shelter?
59.	Dr2:	Definitely. She has nowhere to go if she's not hospitalized. (She
60.		says she will live with her mother or grandmother, but they have
61.		had trouble with her in the past. They both say she can come
62.		home, but wish she could get more treatment. She is not certain
63.		of where she will live.) Her judgment is so poor that even if
64.		she did find someone to take her in, her behavior would get her
65.		evicted in a very short time. (She says she gets four hundred
66.		dollars a month SSI, but she has no idea of how to manage it.
67.		She was hospitalized five months ago with the same problem.)
68.	DA1:	So in your opinion she's gravely disabled?
69.	Dr2:	Yes.
70.	DA1:	And this is because of her mental problems?
71.	Dr2:	Yes. It's the cause of the bad judgment and belligerent
72.		behavior
73.	DA1:	Thank you doctor.
74.	PD3:	In addition to her problem with PCP, is this woman mentally ill?
75.		((silence)) Is this problem a serious mental illness?
76.	Dr2	That's a hard question. In my opinion she also has a bipolar
77.		disorder.
78.	PD3:	Is PCP psychosis an LPS illness, a mental illness? Is it a
79.		serious problem?
80.	Dr2:	Yes combined with the bipolar disorder, it's a very serious
81.		disorder uh illness.
82.	PD3:	So you're convinced that Ms. Farmer is gravely disabled.
83.	Dr2:	That's right.
84.	PD3:	OK, now is the patient oriented to time and place?
85.	Dr2:	Yes.
86.	PD3:	Where has she been living?
87.	Dr2:	She's been living with her grandmother.
88.	PD3:	Does she know her grandmother's phone number?
89.	Dr2:	I think so.
90.	PD3:	Does she know her relatives' names?
91.	Dr2:	Yes.
92.	PD3:	Is she well enough to get home from here by herself?
93.	Dr2:	I suppose so.
94.	PD3:	Can she ride the bus?
95.	Dr2:	Yes.
96.	PD3:	Does she feed and dress herself in the hospital?
97.	Dr2:	As far as I know.
98.	PD3:	Does she understand that it's important to take care of herself,
99.		eat regularly, have a place to stay?
100.	Dr2:	She seems to.
101.	PD3:	Would she go get something to eat if she were hungry?
102.	Dr2:	Yes.

103.	PD3:	So she could take herself down to McDonalds for lunch by
104.		herself?
105.	Dr2:	Yes, I suppose.
106.	J2:	Now I'm not so sure that McDonalds really qualifies as food,
107.		does it Mr. Patrick. [general laughter in courtroom]
108.	PD3:	((laughs)) Arguably. ((silence)) Now doctor, would you say that
109.		Ms. Farmer's symptoms are abating?
110.	Dr2:	Yes, slightly.
111.	PD3:	And why is it, then, that she is unable to provide for her own
112.		food, clothing, and shelter?
113.	Dr2:	She's very confused, delusional, assaultive, threatening. These
114.		things, these behaviors interfere with interpersonal
115.		transactions. She functions very poorly and has poor
116.		reality contact //
117.	PD3:	((breaking in)) What, what delusions has she displayed?
118.	Dr2:	Only the one about being a TV star.
119.	PD3:	But she doesn't have delusions that have anything to do with
120.		food, clothing, or shelter? ((pause)) She isn't afraid of food
121.		for instance?
122.	Dr2:	No, she just has very bad judgment, very confused.
123.	PD3:	That's all, Dr. Fischer. Thank you.
124.	J2:	When you say she's been assaultive, what do you mean, doctor?
125.	Dr2:	She's been very hostile to people she doesn't even know. She
126.		apparently attacked a person in a store, pushed her out the
127.		door. She acts out aggressively in situations where most
128.		people wouldn't react like that.
129.	J2:	How's she been recently?
130.	Dr2:	She's still belligerent. According to her records she's only
131.		been involved in one serious fighting incident on the ward.
132.	J2:	Has her family said that they won't take her back?
133.	Dr2:	They say someone will take her, but they are very reluctant to
134.		stay involved with her if she doesn't show some improvement.
135.	J2:	OK, thank you doctor. Mr. Patrick?
136.	PD3:	We'll call Ms. Farmer.
137.		[Regina Farmer takes the witness stand and is sworn in.]
138.	PD3:	Do you want to leave the hospital, Ms. Farmer?
139.	RF:	Yes I do.
140.	PD3:	Where do you plan to stay?
141.	RF:	With my grandmother or my mother or maybe with my aunt. I
142.		really prefer to stay at my mother's, but I'm not picky. (I
143.		could stay with any of my relatives in town.)
144.	PD3:	How would you support yourself?
145.	RF:	I get SSI.
146.	PD3:	What will you do with your check?
147.	RF:	I'll put it right in the bank. Might take a little cash for
148.		spending items.
149.	PD3:	If you're discharged, how are you going to get around town?

150.	RF:	I guess I'll take the bus.
151.	PD3:	Do you know how to get to your mother's house from here?
152.	RF:	I'm not sure. (If you took me to the bus stop, I could ask the
153.		driver and get a transfer.)
154.	PD3:	Do you know your mother's address?
155.	RF:	3890 Benson street.
156.	PD3:	How about her phone number?
157.	RF:	5 5 5 8 6 4 2. I know how to get there. I'm feeling fine,
158.		// well enough to leave the hospital.
159.	PD3:	((breaking in)) OK now, now if you get out, where are your
160.		clothes and other belongings?
161.	RF:	I have things at my mother's.
162.	PD3:	Are you able to dress yourself all right?
163.	RF:	No problem.
164.	PD3:	What about food? Will you eat if you get hungry?
165.	RF:	Certainly.
166.	PD3:	What would you eat?
167.	RF:	Whatever's in the refrigerator. Or maybe I'd buy a
168.		sandwich or something.
169.	PD3:	Will you be able to cook for yourself?
170.	RF:	I suppose.
171.	PD3:	What would you cook?
172.	RF:	I don't know. Whatever I wanted. Scramble some eggs maybe.
173.		Fix a salad or sandwiches. It's never been a problem.
174.	PD3:	You wouldn't have any trouble getting things to cook?
175.	RF:	I'd shop when I need to.
176.		(PD3 asked several questions regarding shopping for food and
177.		clothing, and what Ms. Farmer would wear. Ms. Farmer said she
178.		knew how to shop and could keep up her wardrobe and dress
179.		herself. PD3 then asked if she would listen to her mother and
180.		grandmother, do what they told her to do, and take her
181.		medications when they told her to. Ms. Farmer agreed that she
182.		would do these things.)
183.	PD3:	Are you going to be able to get along with people?
184.	RF:	I don't see why not, just so they don't bother me.
185.	PD3:	Have you been getting along with these people out in the hall?
186.	RF:	Well enough. They ain't said nothing to me.
187.	PD3:	Do you think it's important to be polite?
188.	RF:	Yes, well, no, not all the time, but usually.
189.	PD3:	How did you get into the hospital?
190.	RF:	The police brought me. They said I was fighting, but it was
191.		only arguing. (Some other woman shoved me so I pushed her
192.		back. The other woman started it, and it was only some
193.		harmless shoving.)
194.	PD3:	Do you use PCP, Regina?
195.	RF:	I did, but I don't now. I never use it on my own. Those

196.		people, my friends, they threatened me to buy that. I don't
197.		use it on my own. I mostly use marijuana.
198.	PD3:	OK Regina. No further questions. ((silence five seconds))
199.	DA1:	How are you doing, Regina?
200.	RF:	Fine. I feel fine.
201.	DA1:	So you've been getting along better with the people at the
202.		hospital?
203.	RF:	I suppose so.
204.	DA1:	What do you think you will do with yourself if you're
205.		discharged?
206.	RF:	I'd like to go back to work. Mind my career.
207.	DA1:	Is that your job on TV?
208.	RF:	That's right.
209.	DA1:	Tell me more about that.
210.	RF:	Well maybe you seen me, seen my show. We've been on for seven
211.		years. I guess you'd say I was the star. (It's hard work
212.		being a TV star. I have to be in front of the camera all day,
213.		and never get a break. I'm very famous and people are always
214.		trying to get my autograph or get me to give them money.) The
215.		Hollywood life is not as glamorous as it seems.
216.	DA1:	Really?
217.	RF:	No, people are always following you around. You never get no
218.		privacy. Everyone in Hollywood knows me.
219.	DA1:	Do you film in Hollywood, which studio?
220.	RF:	I work for all the big studios. I could own them.
221.	DA1:	But which one are you working at now?
222.	RF:	All them producers got to kiss my ass or I'll turn on them.
223.		Without me, they're nothing. They got zip. No star, no show.
224.	DA1:	But when you go to work in the morning, where do you go?
225.	RF:	I go right on the screen. The star is always on screen.
226.	DA1:	((silence three seconds)) Well thank you Ms. Farmer. That's all I
227.		want to ask you.
228.	J2:	I'd like to ask a few questions if I might. ((silence)) Is that
229.		OK with you?
230.	RF:	Sure.
231.	J2:	What is your full name?
232.	RF:	Regina Victoria Farmer.
233.	J2:	Where do you live?
234.	RF:	My mother's house is at 3890 Benson.
235.	J2:	What is your phone number?
236.	RF:	5 5 5 8 6 4 2.
237.	J2:	What is your grandmother's phone number?
238.	RF:	That's 5 5 5 6 7 9 3.
239.	J2:	What's your grandmother's name, Regina?
240.	RF:	Estelle Crawford.
241.	J2:	Who or what are the names of some of your other relatives who

242.　　　　　live in the area?
243.　RF:　My aunt's name is Josephine Williams, and my cousin Janette
244.　　　　　lives with her. ((silence)) You want more?
245.　J2:　No that's fine. Do you know what day it is today?
246.　RF:　Thursday.
247.　J2:　And do you know where you are right now?
248.　RF:　Well I'm in court, Metropolitan Court. ((silence)) I think
249.　　　　　we're down on San Duarte Road somewhere.
250.　J2:　Could you get home from here?
251.　RF:　I said I figure I could get a bus if you showed me where it
252.　　　　　stopped.
253.　J2:　How're you going to do that? Do you know about riding the bus?
254.　RF:　I've done it plenty. You just ask the driver.
255.　J2:　(Judge asks several additional short questions about what Ms.
256.　　　　　Farmer would do if she were released, what she would do if she
257.　　　　　got hungry, what she would wear. Ms. Farmer's replies were
258.　　　　　succinct and responsive.)
259.　J2:　How about your job?
260.　RF:　You mean my acting career? I told you I was a star, didn't I?
261.　　　　　I work in Hollywood.
262.　J2:　Really. Tell me about some of your movies.
263.　RF:　I do mostly TV. It's not as glamorous as you think. It's
264.　　　　　very hard work. Everybody's always demanding things. Do this,
265.　　　　　get over here. I get so tired. I'm thinking about retiring
266.　　　　　anyway since they cancelled my show. I can't get no peace.
267.　　　　　Everybody always wants a piece of you. You don't know who's
268.　　　　　coming and going. (You find that you meet a lot of "friends"
269.　　　　　that you can't trust. People try to get you into trouble.)
270.　　　　　But I don't take that PCP. It's too rough. I just mostly use
271.　　　　　cocaine when I'm shooting a scene. (I really have to take some
272.　　　　　time off to relax.)
273.　J2:　That might be a good idea. That's about it for me. Anything
274.　　　　　else from you Mr. Patrick?
275.　PD3:　Nothing further, your honor. ((silence five seconds)) We just
276.　　　　　don't think Ms. Farmer is gravely disabled your honor. Under
277.　　　　　LPS, involuntary hospitalization should not detain a person
278.　　　　　simply on the basis of being mentally ill. A person can be
279.　　　　　hospitalized only if he can't provide for his own food, clothes,
280.　　　　　and shelter. (I understand the doctor's position and why he thinks
281.　　　　　the patient is mentally ill. I won't argue about the diagnosis.)
282.　　　　　But the symptoms are receding. And more important, they don't
283.　　　　　interfere with Ms. Farmer's providing for her own food, clothes,
284.　　　　　and shelter. If her delusions dealt with food, clothes, and
285.　　　　　shelter, I'd be concerned, but even if she can't stay with her
286.　　　　　mother or grandmother, she can take care of herself. (She can stay
287.　　　　　with other relatives. There are several in the area.) Just

288.		because she's on thin ice with her family is no reason to commit
289.		her. We have lots of people go through here who are on thin ice
290.		with their families, but that's not the basis on which you judge
291.		them. (My client does not meet the criteria for LPS.)
292.		((silence five seconds))
293.	DA1:	This patient has a history of hospitalization and PCP abuse.
294.		She's seriously ill. The doctor is very clear on that and on
295.		the issue of grave disability. Her reality orientation is
296.		poor. She's delusional. Her family wants her to get more
297.		help. She doesn't know what she is going to do and can't
298.		provide for food, clothing, and shelter. That's it.
299.	J2:	How does her mental illness affect her ability to provide for
300.		food, clothes, and shelter?
301.	DA1:	The severeness of her symptoms interferes with her ability to
302.		manage her daily life. (She is so disoriented that she cannot
303.		conduct the routine transactions of everyday life.) If she's
304.		on her own, she will not be able to provide the basic
305.		necessities. She just can't manage the relationships that most
306.		people take for granted.
307.	J2:	She had an altercation in the shopping center. What's this all
308.		about?
309.	DA1:	There was some kind of disturbance and the police arrested her
310.		for being loud and abusive to another shopper.
311.	PD3:	It was some kind of scuffle, your honor, and it's not clear who
312.		was really at fault. She's been much less aggressive since
313.		she's been hospitalized.
314.	DA1:	She's been like this before, your honor. Hospitalized and
315.		released. She doesn't last very long.
316.	J2:	Let me ask you Dr. Fischer, one more time, how does her
317.		mental illness affect her ability to provide food, clothing,
318.		and shelter?
319.	Dr2:	While she says that she's fine, it's just one more example of
320.		her very poor judgment. She may get things arranged for a
321.		time, but her behavior is going to get her into trouble. Her
322.		poor judgment combined with aggressive behavior will make it
323.		impossible to insure that she gets the basic necessities.
324.	J2:	OK. ((silence ten seconds)) I'm going to grant the writ. I
325.		agree with both sides to some extent. I'm concerned with what
326.		appears to be a pattern developing, a pattern of incidents
327.		seems to be emerging. But I'm not prepared to establish the
328.		indignity of grave disability based on the possibility of this
329.		pattern at this time. As long as the family is willing, we'll
330.		give it another try. Can you see to it that she gets in touch
331.		with the mother or the grandmother, Mr. Patrick?
332.	PD3:	As soon as I'm done here.
333.	J2:	OK, let's move along.

Appendix 3:   Patient Jason Andro

[Twenty-two-year old white male, very short (approximately 5 feet 4
inches), neat casual attire, very well groomed]

[Metropolitan Court; J1, DA5, PD4, Dr4]

1.	J1:	Let's do Mr. Andro.
2.	DA5:	May we have Dr. Chin, please. [Witness occupies
3.		witness stand.]
4.	DA5:	Your name please.
5.	Dr4:	Jeffry Chin.
6.	DA5:	Can we stipulate to qualifications?
7.	PD4:	Stipulate.
8.	DA5:	Dr. Chin, do you recognize the man in the green chair?
9.	Dr4:	Yes I do.
10.	DA5:	What is his name?
11.	Dr4:	Jason Andro.
12.	DA5:	How long have you known him?
13.	Dr4:	I've spoken with him several times the past five days.
14.	DA5:	Have you read his chart?
15.	Dr4:	Yes.
16.	DA5:	Have you spoken with others about Mr. Andro?
17.	Dr4:	Yes.
18.	DA5:	And what is your diagnosis.
19.	Dr4:	Mixed organic disorder.
20.	DA5:	Does Mr. Andro have a history of mental disorder.
21.	Dr4:	Yes, his condition appears to go back several years.
22.	DA5:	What fact or facts brought the patient to the hospital this
23.		time?
24.	Dr4:	The police brought him in for fighting with his family. He was
25.		struggling with his sister, pulling her around. He threatened
26.		to kill his mother.
27.	DA5:	And how has his behavior been in the hospital?
28.	Dr4:	He has been very suspicious and demanding. Very delusional.
29.		His delusions have somewhat violent overtones. (He talks about
30.		controlling people and ordering them to do what he says.)
31.	DA5:	In your opinion does his mental illness prevent him from
32.		providing for his own food, clothes, and shelter?
33.	Dr4:	I believe so. He left his job in Tucson to come here where he
34.		had no job. He was arrested for speeding on the freeway while
35.		getting here. (He has been in numerous disputes and incidents
36.		sometimes involving the police. He is constantly antagonizing
37.		people.)
38.	DA5:	Has the patient been placed on medication?
39.	Dr4:	Yes, but there's been minimal improvement. ((silence)) He

40.		doesn't relate at all to other patients on the ward. He
41.		interacts very little with them. He talks frequently with the
42.		nurses but is often incoherent and delusional.
43.	DA5:	Is he delusional during therapy sessions you've had with him?
44.	Dr4:	During treatment he has no insight into his condition, no
45.		recognition of his delusional behavior.
46.	DA5:	So would you conclude that Mr. Andro is gravely disabled.
47.	Dr4:	I would say so.
48.	DA5:	That's all doctor. Thank you.
49.	PD4:	Does Mr. Andro feed and dress himself in the hospital?
50.	Dr4:	Yes.
51.	PD4:	How does he say he will provide for his needs when he leaves
52.		the hospital?
53.	Dr4:	He says he will get a job as a truck driver. He has worked in
54.		various food service jobs but has never worked as a truck
55.		driver.
56.	PD4:	You say that he's improved while in the hospital. Has he had
57.		any fights?
58.	Dr4:	No.
59.	PD4:	Any serious altercations.
60.	Dr4:	No, but he doesn't try to get along with the others.
61.	J1:	In the hospital the man can feed and dress himself. Could he
62.		do this if he were released?
63.	Dr4:	Perhaps if he had a place to stay, someone to help him. But he
64.		doesn't. His family will not take him. He was fighting with
65.		them. He doesn't appear to be able to find a job or manage his
66.		finances because of his mental disorder.
67.	PD4:	That'll be all doctor. Thank you.
68.	J1:	Will we hear from Mr. Andro?
69.	PD4:	Yes your honor, he'd like to testify.
70.		[Jason Andro takes the witness stand and is sworn in.]
71.	PD4:	Mr. Andro, do you want to get out of the hospital?
72.	JA:	Yes ma'am.
73.	PD4:	Can you take care of yourself?
74.	JA:	Yes ma'am.
75.	PD4:	Where would you stay?
76.	JA:	With my parents. Or maybe at a friend's house.
77.	PD4:	Which friend?
78.	JA:	I have a couple in mind. // They've done it before.
79.	PD4:	((breaking in)) Have you been employed?
80.	JA:	Yes, I've done all types of food preparation. You know, working
81.		in restaurants.
82.	PD4:	If you had some money, say four hundred dollars, could you tell
83.		us how you would use it to take care of yourself?
84.	JA:	The first thing I would do would be to buy a car // so I
85.	J1:	((breaking in)) What? Why a car?
86.	JA:	I'd get a car to travel around to find a job.

87.	PD4:	OK now. If you had some money how much would you spend on
88.		rent?
89.	JA:	Nothing if I'm at home. I suppose I should give something if
90.		I crash with a friend though.
91.	PD4:	What about meals?
92.	JA:	I can fix anything. I learned in the restaurants.
93.	PD4:	Would you eat regularly?
94.	JA:	Yes ma'am.
95.	PD4:	Would you take your medications if you were released?
96.	JA:	I guess. ((silence)) Yes ma'am, I'll take it.
97.	PD4:	Will you go to an outpatient program?
98.	JA:	Yes, I've done that before.
99.	PD4:	Do you feel like you've improved since you've been in the
100.		hospital?
101.	JA:	Yes ma'am. One hundred percent // I'm a new man.
102.	PD4:	((breaking in)) Thank you Jason.
103.	DA5:	Do you think you are OK right now?
104.	JA:	Yes ma'am.
105.	DA5:	Tell me why did you quit your job in Tucson?
106.	JA:	I wanted to come and see my family and get a better job here.
107.		In California the pay is better. I was only being paid three
108.		sixty five an hour in Tucson.
109.		(DA5 asks a series of questions about various things that Mr.
110.		Andro has been doing in California. Andro replies that he has
111.		been visiting his family, looking for work and hanging out with
112.		his friends.)
113.	DA5:	Is it true that you heard from your brother before you left
114.		Tucson telling you to come to California?
115.	JA:	Yeah I did.
116.	DA5:	And tell us how you heard from your brother?
117.	JA:	A thing called love. I heard through a thing called love, you
118.		know.
119.	DA5:	A thing called love?
120.	JA:	Yeah you all know what that is.
121.	DA5:	I suppose. When you were admitted to the hospital were you
122.		delusional?
123.	JA:	Yes ma'am, but I'm not now.
124.	DA5:	The doctor says you've been calling yourself Hercules. Why?
125.	JA:	Look at me. I look like Hercules don't I? I am the one.
126.	DA5:	What does that mean?
127.	JA:	You know, the one. The powerful one. You know who I am.
128.	DA5:	Oh?
129.		((silence))
130.	DA5:	Why did the police bring you to the hospital?
131.	JA:	I wasn't really fighting with anyone. I wasn't fighting with
132.		my sister. She was moving my stuff and I was trying to unload

133.		the car to stay there. I wasn't pulling her.
134.	DA5:	Did you say you were going to kill your mother?
135.	JA:	No that's a lie. Others may have made a mistake. I wouldn't
136.		kill nobody.
137.		(After a short silence, DA5 asks a series of questions about
138.		whether Mr. Andro has had altercations with various family
139.		members and friends. Andro denies fighting with any of them,
140.		but admits that he has had several "disagreements.")
141.	DA5:	Haven't you said that your brother is Jesus Christ?
142.	JA:	Yes I think so. Ever since he was born I could see he was
143.		Christ. I guess I saw this when I was about eighteen. About
144.		four years ago.
145.	DA5:	Are you sure?
146.	JA:	As sure as I can be.
147.	DA5:	But didn't you also say that your mother was the devil?
148.	JA:	Yes. I've seen it in her eyes.
149.		((silence))
150.	JA:	It's very difficult with her. Sometimes I find it hard to live
151.		at home.
152.	DA5:	Do you want to live at home now?
153.	JA:	Yes I do. I can do it because I have the power.
154.	DA5:	The power?
155.	JA:	That's right, the power. You know what I mean.
156.	DA5:	That's all Mr. Andro.
157.	J1:	You can go back to your seat now. Ms. Gray?
158.	PD4:	I don't see grave disability here your honor. No income is no
159.		reason to be hospitalized. I'm sure he can find some place to
160.		stay. He seems to think so. He says he's fine and wants to
161.		go.
162.	J1:	Ms. Simmons.
163.	DA5:	Dr. Chin indicates that Mr. Andro is delusional and this will
164.		interfere with carrying out his day-to-day efforts to provide for
165.		himself. (He has no income and no one eager to support him. He
166.		quit a job in order to look for another one in a time of a bad
167.		economy, and that shows very poor judgment. He says he wants to
168.		work in a job that he's never done before. He has no place to stay
169.		and no prospects for finding one. He will have trouble providing
170.		for his food, clothes, and shelter even if he does manage to move in
171.		with someone.) A man his age should be able to support himself and
172.		he can't. His mental illness makes him unemployable. It makes him
173.		unable to take care of himself. People who can take care of
174.		themselves don't say and do the kind of things he does. He seems
175.		to meet every angle of LPS.
176.	J1:	I have to agree. I find Mr. Andro to be gravely disabled. He
177.		is unable at this time to take care of his needs of food,
178.		clothing, and shelter. He is still delusional and can't assume

179.   responsibility for his obligations in the world. He can't get
180.   along with his family, and they are the only ones that seem to
181.   want to have anything to do with him. Let's deny the writ and
182.   remand him for the balance of treatment. This will help you,
183.   Mr. Andro, believe me. ((silence)) Can we do another before
184.   noon?

References

Akers, Ronald. 1972. "Comment on Gove's Evaluation of Societal Reaction as an Explanation of Mental Illness." *American Sociological Review* 37:487–88.

American Psychiatric Association. 1987. *Diagnostic and Statistical Manual of Mental Disorders: DSM-III-R.* Washington, DC: American Psychiatric Association.

Appelbaum, Paul S. and Robert M. Hamm. 1982. "Decisions to Seek Commitment." *Archives of General Psychiatry* 39:447–51.

Appelbaum, Paul S. and Kathleen N. Kemp. 1982. "The Evolution of Commitment Law in the Nineteenth Century." *Law and Human Behavior* 6:343–54.

Atkinson, J. Maxwell and Paul Drew. 1979. *Order in Court.* Atlantic Highlands, NJ: Humanities Press.

Atkinson, J. Maxwell and John C. Heritage. 1984. *Structures of Social Action: Studies in Conversation Analysis.* Cambridge: Cambridge University Press.

Bateson, Gregory, D. Jackson, J. Haley, and J. Weakland. 1956. "Towards a Theory of Schizophrenia." *Behavioral Science* 1:251–64.

Becker, Howard S. 1963. *Outsiders.* New York: Free Press.

Belcher, John R. 1988. "Rights Versus Needs of Homeless Mentally Ill Persons." *Social Work* 33:398–402.

Bell, Leland. V. 1980. *Treating the Mentally Ill: From Colonial Times to the Present.* New York: Praeger.

Bendix, Reinhard. 1960. *Max Weber: An Intellectual Portrait.* New York: Doubleday.

Benson, Paul. 1980. "Labelling Theory and Community Care of the Mentally Ill in California." *Human Organization* 39:134–41.

Berger, Peter L. and Thomas Luckmann. 1966. *The Social Construction of Reality.* Garden City, NY: Doubleday.

Bilmes, Jack. 1986. *Discourse and Behavior.* New York: Plenum.

Bittner, Egon. 1967. "Police Discretion in Emergency Apprehension of Mentally Ill Persons." *Social Problems* 14:278–92.

Bloor, David. 1976. *Knowledge and Social Imagery.* London: Routledge and Kegan Paul.

Blumberg, Abraham S. 1967. *Criminal Justice.* Chicago: Quadrangle.

Blumer, Herbert. 1969. *Symbolic Interactionism*. Berkeley: University of California Press.

Burke, Kenneth. 1950. *A Rhetoric of Motives*. New York: Prentice-Hall.

Bursztajn, Harold, T. Gutheil, M. Mills, R. Hamm, and A. Brodsky. 1986. "Process Analysis of Judges' Commitment Decisions: A Preliminary Empirical Study." *American Journal of Psychiatry* 143:170–74.

Button, Graham and Neil Casey. 1985. "Topic Nomination and Topic Pursuit." *Human Studies* 8:3–55.

Campbell, Richard and Jimmie L. Reeves. 1989. "Covering the Homeless: The Joyce Brown Story." *Critical Studies in Mass Communication* 6:21–42.

Cockerham, William C. 1981. *Sociology of Mental Disorder*. Englewood Cliffs, NJ: Prentice-Hall.

Coulter, Jeff. 1973. *Approaches to Insanity*. New York: Wiley.

———. 1975. "Perceptual Accounts and Interpretive Asymmetries." *Sociology* 9:385–96.

Cousins, Mark and Athar Hussain. 1984. *Michel Foucault*. London: Macmillan.

Decker, Frederic H. 1987. "Psychiatric Management of Legal Defense in Periodic Commitment Hearings." *Social Problems* 34:156–71.

Deutsch, Albert. 1949. *The Mentally Ill in America*, 2nd ed. New York: Columbia University Press.

Dingwall, Robert. 1980. "Orchestrated Encounters." *Sociology of Health and Illness* 2:151–73.

Douglas, Mary. 1986. *How Institutions Think*. Syracuse, NY: Syracuse University Press.

Drew, Paul. 1985. "Analyzing the Use of Language in Courtroom Interaction." Pp. 133–47 in *Handbook of Discourse Analysis*, vol. 3, edited by T. A. van Dijk. London: Academic Press.

Durham, Mary L., Harold D. Carr, and Glenn L. Pierce. 1984. "Police Involvement and Influence in Involuntary Civil Commitment." *Hospital and Community Psychiatry* 35:580–84.

Durkheim, Emile. 1961. *The Elementary Forms of the Religious Life*. New York: Collier-Macmillan.

Emerson, Robert M. 1969. *Judging Delinquents*. Chicago: Aldine.

———. 1981. "On Last Resorts." *American Journal of Sociology* 87:1–22.

———. 1983. "Holistic Effects in Social Control Decision-making." *Law and Society Review* 17:425–55.

———. 1989. "Tenability and Troubles: The Construction of Accommodative Relations by Psychiatric Emergency Teams." Pp. 215–37 in *Perspectives on Social Problems*, vol. 1, edited by J. Holstein and G. Miller. Greenwich, CT: JAI Press.

Emerson, Robert M. and Sheldon L. Messinger. 1977. "The Micro-politics of Trouble." *Social Problems* 25:121–34.

Felman, Shoshana. 1985. *Writing and Madness*. Ithaca, NY: Cornell University Press.

Foucault, Michel. 1965. *Madness and Civilization*. New York: Random House.

———. 1972. *The Archaeology of Knowledge*. New York: Pantheon.

———. 1973. *The Birth of the Clinic*. New York: Random House.

————. 1987. *Mental Illness and Psychology*. Berkeley: University of California Press.

Gallagher, Bernard J. 1987. *The Sociology of Mental Illness*. Englewood Cliffs, NJ: Prentice-Hall.

Garfinkel, Harold. 1967. *Studies in Ethnomethodology*. Englewood Cliffs, NJ: Prentice-Hall.

Garfinkel, Harold and Harvey Sacks. 1970. "On Formal Structures of Practical Actions." Pp. 338–66 in *Theoretical Sociology*, edited by J. C. McKinney and E. A. Tiryakian. New York: Appleton Century Crofts.

Gerson, Judith M. and Kathy Peiss. 1985. "Boundaries, Negotiation, Consciousness: Reconceptualizing Gender Relations." *Social Problems* 32:317–31.

Gibbs, Jack and M. Erickson. 1975. "Major Developments in the Sociological Study of Deviance." *Annual Review of Sociology* 1:21–42.

Giddens, Anthony. 1971. *Capitalism and Modern Social Theory*. Cambridge: Cambridge University Press.

————. 1979. *Central Problems in Social Theory*. Berkeley: University of California Press.

Gilboy, Janet A. and John R. Schmidt. 1971. "Voluntary Hospitalization of the Mentally Ill." *Northwestern Law Review* 66:429–40.

Goffman, Erving. 1961. *Asylums*. Garden City, NY: Doubleday.

————. 1969. "The Insanity of Place." *Psychiatry* 32:357–88.

Gove, Walter R. 1970. "Societal Reaction as an Explanation of Mental Illness: An Evaluation. American Sociological Review. 35:873-84.

————. 1975. "The Labelling Theory of Mental Illness: A Reply to Scheff." *American Sociological Review* 40:242–48.

————. 1976. "Reply to Imershein and Simons and Scheff." *American Sociological Review* 41:564–67.

————. 1980a. "The Labelling Perspective: An Overview." Pp. 9–25 in *The Labelling of Deviance: Evaluating a Perspective*, 2nd ed., edited by W. Gove. Beverly Hills: Sage.

————. 1980b. "Labelling and Mental Illness: A Critique." Pp. 53–99 in *The Labelling of Deviance: Evaluating a Perspective*, 2nd ed., edited by W. Gove. Beverly Hills: Sage.

———— 1982. "The Current Status of the Labelling Theory of Mental Illness." Pp. 273–300 in *Deviance and Mental Illness*, edited by W. Gove. Beverly Hills: Sage.

Greenley, James R. 1972. "The Psychiatric Patient's Family and Length of Hospitalization." *Journal of Health and Social Behavior* 13:25–37.

Gubrium, Jaber F. 1987. "Organizational Embeddedness and Family Life." Pp. 23–41 in *Aging, Health, and Family: Long Term Care*, edited by T. Brubaker. Newbury Park, CA: Sage.

————. 1988. *Analyzing Field Reality*. Newbury Park, CA: Sage.

————. 1989. "Local Cultures and Service Policy." Pp. 94–112 in *The Politics of Field Research*, edited by J. Gubrium and D. Silverman. London: Sage.

————. 1991. "Recognizing and Analyzing Local Cultures." Pp. 131–41 in *Experiencing Fieldwork*, edited by W. Shaffir and R. Stebbins. Newbury Park, CA: Sage.

————. 1992. *Out of Control.* Newbury Park, CA: Sage.

Gubrium, Jaber F. and James. A. Holstein. 1990. *What Is Family?* Mt. View, CA: Mayfield.

————. 1993. *Constructing the Life Course.* New York: General Hall.

Haney, C. Allen and Robert Michielutte. 1968. "Selective Factors Operating in the Adjudication of Incompetency." *Journal of Health and Social Behavior* 9:233–42.

Haney, C. Allen, Kent S. Miller, and Robert Michielutte. 1969. "The Interaction of Petitioner and Deviant Social Characteristics in the Adjudication of Incompetency." *Sociometry* 32:182–93.

Hasenfeld, Yeheskel. 1972. "People Processing Organizations: An Exchange Approach." *American Sociological Review* 37:256–63.

Heritage, John C. 1983. "Accounts in Action." Pp. 117–31 in *Accounts and Action,* edited by N. Gilbert and P. Abell. Farnborough, UK: Gower.

————. 1984. *Garfinkel and Ethnomethodology.* Cambridge: Cambridge University Press.

Hiday, Virginia A. 1983. "Judicial Decisions in Civil Commitment: Facts, Attitudes, and Psychiatric Recommendations." *Law and Society Review* 17:517–30.

————. 1988. "Civil Commitment: A Review of Empirical Research." *Behavioral Sciences and the Law* 6:15–43.

Hollingshead, Agust B. and Frederick C. Redlich. 1958. *Social Class and Mental Illness.* New York: Wiley.

Holstein, James A. 1983. "Jurors' Use of Judges' Instructions: Conceptual and Methodological Issues for Simulated Jury Research." *Sociological Methods and Research* 11:501–18.

————. 1984. "The Placement of Insanity: Assessments of Grave Disability and Involuntary Commitment Decisions." *Urban Life* 13:35–62.

————. 1987a. "Producing Gender Effects on Involuntary Mental Hospitalization." *Social Problems* 34:141–55.

————. 1987b. "Mental Illness Assumptions in Civil Commitment Proceedings." *Journal of Contemporary Ethnography* 16:147–75.

————. 1988a. "Court Ordered Incompetence: Conversational Organization in Involuntary Commitment Hearings." *Social Problems* 35:458–73.

————. 1988b. "Studying 'Family Usage': Family Image and Discourse in Mental Hospitalization Decisions." *Journal of Contemporary Ethnography* 17:261–84.

————. 1990a. "The Discourse of Age in Involuntary Commitment Proceedings." *Journal of Aging Studies* 4:111–130.

————. 1990b. "Describing Home Care: Discourse and Image in Involuntary Commitment Proceedings." Pp. 209–26 in *The Home Care Experience,* edited by J. Gubrium and A. Sankar. Newbury Park, CA: Sage.

————. 1992. "Producing People: Descriptive Practice in Human Service Work." Pp. 23–39 in *Current Research on Occupations and Professions,* edited by G. Miller. Greenwich, CT: JAI Press.

Horwitz, Allan V. 1979. "Models, Muddles, and Mental Illness Labeling." *Journal of Health and Social Behavior* 20:296–300.

————. 1982. *The Social Control of Mental Illness.* New York: Academic Press.

Imershein, Allen W. and Ronald L. Simons. 1976. "Rules and Examples in Lay and Professional Psychiatry: An Ethnomethodological Comment on the Scheff-Gove Controversy." *American Sociological Review* 41:559–63.

Kessler, Ronald C. and Paul D. Cleary. 1980. "Social Class and Psychological Distress." *American Sociological Review* 45:463–78.

Kirk, Stuart. and M. E. Thierren. 1975. "Community Mental Health Myths and the Fate of Former Hospitalized Patients." *Psychiatry* 38:209–17.

Kitsuse, John I. 1962. "Societal Reactions to Deviant Behavior: Problems of Theory and Method." *Social Problems* 9:247–56.

————. 1980. "The 'New Conception of Deviance' and Its Critics." Pp. 381–92 in *The Labelling of Deviance,* edited by W. Gove. Beverly Hills: Sage.

Krohn, Marvin and Ronald L. Akers. 1977. "An Alternative View of the Labeling Versus Psychiatric Perspectives on Societal Reaction to Mental Illness." *Social Forces* 56:341–62.

Kutner, Luis. 1962. "The Illusion of Due Process in Commitment Proceedings." *Northwestern University Law Review* 57:383–99.

Laing, R.D. 1967. *The Politics of Experience.* New York: Pantheon.

Laing, R.D. and A. Esterson. 1964. *Sanity, Madness and the Family.* London: Tavistock.

Levenson, James L. 1986. "Psychiatric Commitment and Involuntary Hospitalization: An Ethical Perspective." *Psychiatric Quarterly* 58:106–12.

Lewis, Dan A., Edward Goetz, Mark Schoenfield, Andrew C. Gordon, and Eugene Griffin. 1984. "The Negotiation of Involuntary Civil Commitment." *Law and Society Review* 18:629–49.

Linsky, Arnold S. 1970a. "Community Homogeneity and Exclusion of the Mentally Ill: Rejection vs. Consensus About Deviance." *Journal of Health and Social Behavior* 11:304–11.

————. 1970b. "Who Shall Be Excluded: The Influence of Personal Attributes in Community Reaction to the Mentally Ill." *Social Psychiatry* 5:166–71.

Lipsky, Michael. 1980. *Street-Level Bureaucracy.* New York: Russell Sage Foundation.

Loseke, Donileen R. 1989. "Creating Clients: Social Problems Work in a Shelter for Battered Women. Pp. 173–194 in *Perspectives on Social Problems,* vol. 1, edited by J. Holstein and G. Miller. Greenwich, CT: JAI Press.

————. 1992. *The Battered Woman and Shelters.* Albany, NY: SUNY Press.

Lynch, Michael. 1983. "Accommodation Practices: Vernacular Treatments of Madness." *Social Problems* 31:152–63.

Maynard, Douglas W. 1980. "Placement of Topic Changes in Conversation." *Semiotica* 30:263–90.

————. 1984. *Inside Plea Bargaining.* New York: Plenum.

Mechanic, David. 1980. *Mental Health and Social Policy.* Englewood Cliffs, NJ: Prentice-Hall.

Mehan, Hugh. 1979. *Learning Lessons.* Cambridge, MA: Harvard University Press.

Mestrovic, Stjepan. 1983. "Need for Treatment and New York's Revised Commitment Laws." *International Journal of Law and Psychiatry* 6:75–88.

Miller, Dorothy and Michael Schwartz. 1966. "County Lunacy Commission Hearings: Some Observations of Commitments to a State Mental Hospital." *Social Problems* 14:26–35.

Miller, Gale. 1990. "Work as Reality Maintaining Activity: Interactional Aspects of Occupational and Professional Work." Pp. 163–83 in *Current Research on Occupations and Professions,* vol. 5, edited by H. Lopata. Greenwich, CT: JAI Press.

———. 1991. *Enforcing the Work Ethic.* Albany, NY: SUNY Press.

Miller, Gale and James A. Holstein. 1989. "On The Sociology of Social Problems." Pp. 1–16 in *Perspectives on Social Problems,* vol. 1, edited by J. Holstein and G. Miller. Greenwich, CT: JAI Press.

Miller, Robert D., Rebecca Maher, and Paul B. Fiddleman. 1984. "The Use of Plea Bargaining in Civil Commitment." *International Journal of Law and Psychiatry* 7:395–406.

Mills, C. Wright. 1940. "Situated Actions and Vocabularies of Motive." *American Sociological Review* 5:904–13.

Mollica, Richard F. 1983. "From Asylum to Community: The Threatened Disintegration of Public Psychiatry." *New England Journal of Medicine* 308:367–73.

Morrissey, Joseph P. and Howard H. Goldman. 1984. "Cycles of Reform in the Care of the Chronically Mentally Ill." *Hospital and Community Psychiatry* 35:785–793.

Morse, Stephen J. 1982. "A Preference for Liberty: The Case Against Involuntary Commitment of the Mentally Disordered." Pp. 69–109 in *The Court of Last Resort,* by C. Warren. Chicago: University of Chicago Press.

Nicholson, Robert A. 1986. "Correlates of Commitment Status in Psychiatric Patients." *Psychological Bulletin* 100:241–50.

Pollner, Melvin. 1974. "Sociological and Common Sense Models of the Labeling Process." Pp. 27–40 in *Ethnomethodology,* edited by R. Turner. Middlesex, UK: Penguin.

———. 1975. "'The Very Coinage of Your Brain': The Anatomy of Reality Disjunctures." *Philosophy of the Social Sciences* 5:411–30.

———. 1978. "Constitutive and Mundane Versions of Labeling Theory." *Human Studies* 1:269–288.

———. 1987. *Mundane Reason.* Cambridge: Cambridge University Press.

Rosenfield, Sarah. 1984. "Race Differences in Involuntary Hospitalization: Psychiatric vs. Labelling Perspectives." *Journal of Health and Social Behavior* 25:14–23.

Rosenhan, David L. 1973. "On Being Sane in Insane Places." *Science* 179:250–58.

Rothman, David J. 1971. *The Discovery of the Asylum.* Boston: Little, Brown.

Rushing, William A. 1971. "Individual Resources, Societal Reaction, and Hospital Commitment." *American Journal of Sociology* 77:511–26.

Sacks, Harvey. 1972. "An Initial Investigation of the Usability of Conversational Data for Doing Sociology." Pp. 31–75 in *Studies in Social Interaction,* edited by D. Sudnow. New York: Free Press.

Sacks, Harvey and Emanuel Schegloff. 1979. "Two Preferences in the Organization of Reference to Persons in Conversation and Their Interaction." Pp. 15–

21 in *Everyday Language Studies in Ethnomethodology*, edited by G. Psathas. New York: Irvington.

Sacks, Harvey, Emanuel Schegloff, and Gail Jefferson. 1974. "A Simplest Systematics for the Organization of Turn-taking for Conversation." *Language* 50:696–735.

Sagarin, Edward and F. Montanino. 1976. "Anthologies and Readers on Deviance." *Contemporary Sociology* 5:259–67.

Scheff, Thomas J. 1964. "The Societal Reaction to Deviance: Ascriptive Elements in the Psychiatric Screening of Mental Patients in a Midwestern State." *Social Problems* 11:401–13.

_____. 1966. *Being Mentally Ill*. Chicago: Aldine.

_____. 1967. "Social Conditions for Rationality: How Urban and Rural Courts Deal with the Mentally Ill." *American Behavioral Scientist* 7:21–27.

_____. 1974. "The Labelling Theory of Mental Illness." *American Sociological Review* 39:444–52.

_____. 1975. "Reply to Chauncey and Gove." *American Sociological Review* 40:252–57.

_____. 1976. "Reply to Imershein and Simons." *American Sociological Review* 41:563–64.

Schegloff, Emanuel A. 1982. "Discourse as an Interactional Achievement: Some Uses of 'Uh huh' and Other Things That Come Between Sentences." Pp. 71–93 in *Georgetown University Roundtable on Language and Linguistics*, edited by D. Tannen. Washington, DC: Georgetown University Press.

_____. 1987. "Analyzing Single Episodes of Interaction: An Exercise in Conversation Analysis." *Social Psychology Quarterly* 50:101-14.

Schlossman, Steven L. 1977. *Love and the American Delinquent*. Chicago: University of Chicago Press.

Schutz, Alfred. 1962. *The Problem of Social Reality*. The Hague: Martinus Nijhoff.

_____. 1964. *Studies in Social Theory*. The Hague: Martinus Nijhoff.

_____. 1970. *On Phenomenology and Social Relations*. Chicago: University of Chicago Press.

Scott, R.D. 1974. "Cultural Frontiers in the Mental Health Service." *Schizophrenia Bulletin* 10:58–73.

Scull, Andrew. 1981. "A New Trade in Lunacy." *American Behavioral Scientist* 24:741–54.

Shuman, Daniel W. 1985. "Innovative Statutory Approaches to Civil Commitment: An Overview and Critique." *Law, Medicine, and Health Care* 13:284–89.

Smith, Dorothy E. 1978. "'K' is Mentally Ill: The Anatomy of a Factual Account." *Sociology* 12:23–53.

Smith, Steven R. and Robert G. Meyer. 1987. *Law, Behavior, and Mental Health*. New York: New York University Press.

Snow, David, S. Baker, L. Anderson, and M. Martin. 1986. "The Myth of Pervasive Mental Illness Among the Homeless." *Social Problems* 33:407–23.

Steadman, Henry and Joseph H. Cocozza. 1974. *Careers of the Criminally Insane*. Lexington, MA: Lexington Books.

Stoffelmayr, Bertram, David Roth, William Parker, and Dale Dillavou. 1988. "Legal Status and Patient Behavior at the Time of Hospitalization." *American Journal of Forensic Psychology* 1:5–14.

Szasz, Thomas. S. 1961. *The Myth of Mental Illness.* New York: Harper.

Thomas, W.I. 1931. *The Unadjusted Girl.* Boston: Little, Brown.

Thompson, Judith S. and Joel W. Ager. 1988. "An Experimental Analysis of the Civil Commitment Recommendations of Psychologists and Psychiatrists." *Behavioral Sciences and the Law* 6:119–29.

Vandewater, Steven R. 1983. "Discourse Processes and the Social Organization of Group Therapy Sessions." *Sociology of Health and Illness* 5:275–96.

Warren, Carol A. B. 1977. "Involuntary Commitment for Mental Disorder: The Application of California's Lanterman-Petris-Short Act." *Law and Society Review* 11:629–49.

———. 1981. "New Forms of Social Control: The Myth of Deinstitutionalization." *American Behavioral Scientist* 24:724–40.

———. 1982. *The Court of Last Resort.* Chicago: University of Chicago Press.

Weber, Max. 1958. *The Protestant Ethic and the Spirit of Capitalism.* New York: Scribners.

———. 1968. *Economy and Society.* New York: Bedminster Press.

Wenger, Dennis L. and C. Richard Fletcher. 1969. "The Effect of Legal Counsel on Admissions to a State Mental Hospital: A Confrontation of Professions." *Journal of Health and Social Behavior* 10:66–72.

West, Candace. 1984. *Routine Complications: Troubles with Talk Between Doctors and Patients.* Bloomington: Indiana University Press.

Wexler, David B. 1988. "Reforming the Law in Action Through Empirically Grounded Civil Commitment Guidelines." *Hospital and Community Psychiatry* 39:402-405.

Wilde, William A. 1968. "Decision-making in A Psychiatric Screening Agency." *Journal of Health and Social Behavior* 9:215–21.

Zimmerman, Don H. 1970. "The Practicalities of Rule Use." Pp. 221–38 in *Understanding Everyday Life,* edited by J. Douglas. Chicago: Aldine.

Zimmerman, Don H. and D. Lawrence Wieder. 1970. "Ethnomethodology and the Problem of Order." Pp. 287–98 in *Understanding Everyday Life,* edited by J. Douglas. Chicago: Aldine.

Index

217